THE
THIN
COMMANDMENTS

Robert Simms

ISBN: 978-0-9858233-6-8
Printed in the United States of America

CONTENTS

1
Returning to the Original Commandments
The Strategy for this Book

Some years ago I developed a poster I called *The Thin Commandments*. I came up with the idea independently, but I soon discovered that a number of other people had also lit on the same idea of comparing their chosen weight loss strategies to the Ten Commandments of biblical fame. At least, they adapted their *title* from those famous, divine utterances; in looking at the various Thin Commandments available out there on the market, the reader can readily see that the resemblance of each list to the Ten Commandments pretty much ends at the name.

For instance, there's *The Thin Commandments: The Ten No-Fail Strategies for Permanent Weight Loss,* by Stephen Gullo, a book listing ten overarching rules for successful dieting, including: "Think historically, not just calorically," "Identify trigger foods that can undermine your weight loss," "Slips should teach you, not defeat you," etc.

"Thin Commandments," an article about eating disorders by Angie Best-Boss, reviews another book, *The Thin*

Commandments, by Carolyn Costin, aimed at folks with eating disorders. Costin's tongue-in-cheek commandments aren't meant to be followed but to illustrate beliefs that lead people astray. Unfortunately, they have been embraced as serious goals by "pro-ana" folks—which stands for "pro-anorexic." Those maxims include: 1) If you aren't thin, you aren't attractive... 2) Being thin is more important than being healthy... and 4) Thou shall not eat without feeling guilty. In the same vein, "The Thin Commandments," a film by Darryl Roberts, critiques the diet craze and those who promote unhealthy skinniness.

Another list of Commandments was devised by Ellen Foster for a magazine article. It handed down the following ten:

1. Find six things you can change without screaming.
2. Don't eat raw food after 4PM.
3. Eat every meal super slowly.
4. Break the TV = Treat Time habit.
5. Throw out your microwave.
6. Take a pro-biotic supplement.
7. Never start a diet on a Monday.
8. Eat like a cave woman.
9. Remember: not all calories are equal.
10. Imagine food and you'll eat less of it.

The article represented itself as a compendium of the best weight loss tips from nutritional experts. Some good advice can be gleaned from these commandments, but they're disparate strategies drawn from differing theories of nutrition, and as such they lack a cohesive philosophy that the average person can grasp. In addition, if all followed, they would created an almost bizarre lifestyle. Not to mention that they are in conflict with each other: you can't eat like a cave woman (never eat anything a cave woman wouldn't recognize) and consume pro-biotics at the same time.

Other lists of rules

While a few diet experts have popularized their systems by picking up on the "thin commandments" concept, diet authorities have long issued lists of rules without trying to sound cute or innovative. These lists are always reflections of the values, opinions, experiences, impressions, knowledge, and also mis-impressions, mistaken conclusions and prejudices of their creators. Most of us don't know as much as any of the experts do, and many of us don't even know as much as the self-proclaimed but not verified experts do, so we don't know how to tell if their lists are really based on impeccable science and are proven to be profoundly helpful.

What *would* help would be for their lists to relate to the average person and to be simple to follow. Unfortunately, they often sound more like they were addressed to other nutritionists instead of the rest of us.

Here's a list from Ellen Seidman, in News&Views on Health.com:

1. Load up on low-glycemic foods

2. Eat more protein-rich foods
3. Don't worry so much about full-fat dairy
4. Balance your meals
5. Quit obsessing over calories[1]

The list starts off disappointingly, since most people have no idea what glycemic means, much less how to get less of such foods. Rule 2 is a bit less obscure, since most of us think, "Protein—oh, that's meat!" Yes, it is, but protein isn't limited to meat. The rest of the suggestions aren't bad at all. I will discuss in upcoming pages the matter of full-fat dairy, which is butter and whole milk, etc. "Balanced meals" sounds like it refers to meat, vegetables and fruits, but Seidman's explanation again goes into nutritional jargon. However, she finishes on a high note about not being overly concerned with calories, with which I agree wholeheartedly.

The list, however, lacks a unifying theme. Certainly it isn't inspirational, and if there's one thing every person who has ever gone on a diet knows, we need inspiration! That's one reason I developed my concept of the *Thin Commandments.* I wanted to provide myself, and eventually others, with an inspirational way of looking at a challenge that many of us face.

This is not that.
This book does not follow any of the above approaches to

---

[1]Ellen Seidman, "5 Really Simple New Rules for Weight Loss," *Health* (May 19, 2015), *http://news.health.com/2015/05/19/5-really-simple-new-rules-for-weight-loss,* Accessed March 29, 2015.

losing weight and maintaining a healthy target mass. The theory I followed in creating my *Thin Commandments* was to return to the original TEN COMMANDMENTS—not just the name, and not a superficial or whimsical similarity to them, but to the concepts articulated in those Commandments. Specifically, I studied the original commandments given to Moses on Mount Sinai, with the purpose of adapting them to the challenge many people face of losing weight. My guiding question was, Can the Ten Commandments be restated, retaining their biblical force and meaning, with a specific application to weight loss? I believe they can, and I present the resulting *Thin Commandments* in this book.

The Ten Commandments can be restated with a specific application to weight loss.

I took this approach not as a novelty, as one might if he had only a passing acquaintance with the original Ten Commandments. By profession I am a judge, but for twenty five years I was a Christian pastor and I still preach as well as write on biblical subjects. I come to the Ten Commandments of the Bible with the deepest reverence and quite a bit of learning. In studying them with this purpose in mind, I was fundamentally interested in extracting the profound purposes of the Commandments and then applying their lessons to this narrow subject that engages all of us: food.

The plan of this book is simple. First, I'm going to give you an overview of the basic weakness in most approaches to dieting, and a summation of the theory behind the approach that avoids all those weaknesses. Then we'll look at the *Thin Commandments* themselves.

Right off the bat, I want you to understand that you will get no recipes, no calorie counters, and no lists of common and wonderful things to stop eating or strange and tasteless foods to start consuming. This book *reasons* with you about things that should be self- evident to all of us but that most of us are prone to losing sight of. This book is about values, the kind that enrich your spiritual life and your relationships with others, as well as helping you develop a sound view of your own worth, both in God's eyes and your own.

2
The Road to Fat was Indulgence;
The Road to Slim is Discipline

D o not, *do not*, let the title to this chapter offend you. Do not decide that the rest of this book is going to give you a verbal spanking or lay a guilt trip on you. It isn't. I just believe in calling fat what it is, and in being candid about the core philosophy that will enable you to succeed in this matter that you believe is of critical importance. If you didn't think that losing that extra weight of yours was extremely important, you wouldn't have bought this book. So open your mind and heart, and reconsider what the title prepares you for: you gained weight by *indulging*—in all likelihood just a little now and then, but it all added up. If you're going to reverse the course of your weight and be slim again, or slim for the first time, you're going to have to increase your level of *discipline.*

Fortunately, you're already disciplined about some things in your life—I know you are. You may get up and go to work every day at a specific time. You drive a car and you obey the rules of the road (most of the time!). You pay your bills. You observe the rules of this and that, and you may have a hobby or other activity that you make time for or carry out with regularity. All these things require and make use of discipline. What you need to do is not to acquire some skill you *don't* have, but to exercise and increase your strength in a skill you *do* have, so as to meet the challenge ahead of you.

Unfortunately, dieting (that's an off-putting word, isn't it?) invites the temptation to find an easy way out, a fast way through. We conclude immediately, whether rightly or wrongly, that a diet will be painful and thoroughly unenjoyable, and we look for some strategy that promises a miracle cure or a shortcut.

Let me illustrate. In the face of the seeming impossibility of traveling to other solar systems or even other galaxies because of the daunting distances, astrophysicists theorize that it may be possible to employ a shortcut called a worm hole, a phenomenon that might exist if space-time is folded or rolled on itself. A ship might enter one end of the worm hole, travel in it ever so briefly, and exit many light years away. Wouldn't it be wonderful to have that sort of means of getting from the weight you are right now to the weight you'd like to be, in no time at all, even though the distance in terms of pounds may be significant? I know the feeling. We want to skip the difficulties and the time, and undo the past in a moment.

One of the things we most hope to avoid about dieting is having to exercise will power. The immensely popular Dr. Phil McGraw, a psychologist by profession previous to being just Dr. Phil, a counselor of television fame, was interviewed on Fox News in 2015 about weight loss. When asked what he thought about the old standard recommendation of will power he said that will power doesn't work and wasn't necessary. What you have to do, opined Dr. Phil, is surround yourself with people who will encourage and help you. That was his assessment of will power, which, to the contrary, I insist is a necessary component to any and every diet strategy a person may ever try.

Where Dr. Phil got the idea that will power isn't necessary, I don't know. Maybe he and I have different definitions for the term. He may be talking about some nearly supernatural strength to radically change almost everything in your life, a revolution astounding not only everyone around you but you, yourself. Or, he may be talking about that sort of painful self-denial that robs you of daily enjoyment and makes you bad company, a herculean effort sustained only by gritting your teeth and turning down every pleasure set in front of you.

Thankfully, and beneficially for you, my definition is straightforward: will power is the force of one's will to accomplish a purpose. It's the determination to do the things necessary to succeed in that purpose, against casual loss of commitment and against temptations to quit or inducements to give in. I maintain that without this will power, an army of people cheering you on won't be able to keep you from defying their encouragement by quitting. Apart from your being captured and confined and fed a slimming diet by guards who cannot be bribed to give you more, whatever diet plan you choose will require you to stick to it, in a world where food is readily available in mass quantities. Will power is not the only thing you need to lose weight, but a measure of it is essential.

However, will power is not stern negativism. It's merely the thing I've just told you that you already possess, because another word for will power is *discipline*. There really is no way to avoid the fact that for diets to be permanently successful you must employ a component of discipline. The good news is that you already have this innate capacity for discipline: you probably just need to tone it up.

THE WEAKNESSES OF DIETS

Many people have dieted using methods promoted as easy, and some people will swear by those methods and argue with my assertion about discipline. Let's look at the "easy" options, the ways people try to make short cuts or worm holes to weight loss. Then we'll narrow our focus and identify the most reasonable, most successful, most sustainable method of losing weight.

1. Diet Foods

A few diet plans call principally for the consumption of diet foods as their strategy to lose weight. By "diet foods" I mean foods that are not only low in calories but that are also specially developed to be so, in order to provide dieters with something they can eat to their hearts' content without excessively running up their caloric intake. Diet foods include anything artificially sweetened such as: sodas and some packed fruits or juices; anything you artificially sweeten yourself such as coffee or tea with saccharin, aspartame or sorbitol; sugar free candy and sugar free syrup (these almost defy their names), and a host of innovations in food that contain ingredients that give them bulk without much in the way of calories.

The problem with diet foods is first that it is not reasonable to expect that people will continue to consume them the rest of their lives. Dieting is about reaching a target weight and then maintaining it, and maintaining target weight requires a lower caloric intake than maintaining your pre-diet weight. If you depend on diet foods to keep your caloric intake lower while not adjusting the amount of food you eat, you will have to eat diet foods for the rest of your life to succeed. The problem with that is that diet foods are not, by their nature, very satisfying.

I know that various diet food makers advertise their products by claiming the opposite, that their foods actually taste rich and sinful! If you have tasted them, you know the claims are hype. Unless you have no taste buds, or you have some disease that has taken away your sense of taste (and probably smell, as well, which is related), you will not think that diet foods, by and large, are really tasty. Possibly you have never had quality food to begin with, in which case diet foods may be as tasty as anything you've ever had. But if you know the taste of chicken Parmesan made from a genuine Italian recipe, for instance, the Weight Watchers®

version is going to have very little taste at all, by comparison. Same with cheese. Processed cheese food substitutes or fake cheese made with nothing but some esoteric oil cannot hold a candle to real cheese.

I know people who limit their calories by eating some imitation of the real thing, and they tell me with pride, "I've gotten to where I like it just as much." Clearly they haven't had the real thing in quite a while and have forgotten what it tastes like. And if they've really come to the point at which they think the imitation is just as good, I think it's sad.

Puffed rice cakes are another good example of diet foods. When these pieces of fluffy nothing began to proliferate in stores and appear in various flavors to keep the interest of dieters everywhere, a friend of mine described them as "ghost food." I tried them once or twice and found them not to be very interesting. They gave my mouth something to do, but there was no satisfaction in them at all. It occurred to me that if the point is merely to give your mouth an engaging activity, your weight problem is likely due to your oral habit, like a smoker who tries to quit and has to chew gum.

Many if not most other diet foods are bland, tasteless, or the opposite—having a chemical taste—and not palatable for the long term. Across the board, artificial sweeteners, for instance, are bitter or have an aftertaste. Some people say they get used to them and cannot tell the difference between tea or sodas with artificial sweeteners and the same beverages sweetened with sugar. This is more of a comment on the sensitivity of these people to various tastes than anything else, and again, it's somewhat sad that they cannot distinguish these tastes. Surely the solution to the dieter's challenge is not to get used to tasteless foods.

Further, diet foods often make use of chemicals that may have long term effects that are less than beneficial. Now, I don't have an aversion to the idea that my food may contain "chemicals." Technically, all substances are chemicals. I took quite a lot of chemistry classes in college and I know how to make a number of common flavors in the laboratory. But some of the things diet food makers employ to give their creations the consistency of the genuine article, or to

---

Surely the solution to the dieter's challenge is not to get used to tasteless foods.

---

sweeten or salt them, or to add some texture, may have long term effects we don't yet know about.

Even the short term effects that are known may be something to avoid. For instance, Olestra is an oil substitute used in some high fat foods, such as potato chips. It doesn't have the impact on LDL cholesterol that some fats do, and in fact, it tends to go through the digestive system without having much effect at all nutritionally. This, in fact, is the reason its main side effect is that if you eat a lot of those chips because you think they won't hurt you, the Olestra *runs* right through you and, well, you can figure out the rest.

Years ago when my wife would buy some food loaded with all sorts of hard-to-pronounce chemicals to make it smell, taste and chew like the real thing, I told her I didn't want to dine on butylated hydroxy toluene. That's a real chemical, by the way; it's known as BHT, and it's a preservative. I started using the chemical name as an all purpose adjective for any complex chemical used in making diet foods. As I say, I have no aversion to time tested preservatives; it's the fake food ingredients I prefer to skip. I'm not so much scared that they will give me cancer as I am opposed to their simply not being the real foods that God made to grow in the ground, hang on the trees, swim in the water or congregate in the barnyard.

2. Fad Diets

Fad diets are those contrived diet plans that feature odd foods or a severely limited number of foods, often put together in unusual combinations, requiring the dieter to follow stringent intake rules for a certain number of days or weeks in order to see dramatic progress. One such fad diet is The Rotation Diet, developed by Martin Katahn. It involves eating precisely prescribed meals for a first week, another set of specific meals for a second week, and so on, for four weeks, followed by a return to what is essentially the first week with some variation, and continuing through eight weeks. At the end of the eight weeks, the plan may be repeated.

Without going into the theory, I may say, from personal experience no less, that The Rotation Diet works, in that you do lose weight. However, it requires picky grocery shopping and great attention to weighing foods in precise ounces and counting crackers and measuring liquids, etcetera, and generally becomes a tedious project. It's novel, and can be interesting for a while, but as a lifestyle it would be strange. It consumes your attention (pun intended) and becomes your life for the duration. Furthermore, if you're not the only person in your household, such a diet either requires everyone else to be on it or for you to do your own cooking—or to expect the person who *does* cook to prepare two meals. It's not simple to go through this diet.

Of course, The Rotation Diet, as any other fad diet, is not meant to be continued for life; you lose the weight you want by using the diet and then you get off it. It's when you get off it that you face the underlying challenge: eating differently than you used to. Further, The Rotation Diet's recommendations for maintenance attempt to convince you to eat different foods—eliminating this and including that—for the rest of your life. You may or may not find its recommendations palatable.

In spite of the inclusion in the typical fad diet's instructions of admonitions to change your way of eating, no fad diet really gives you significant help in making these adjustments. That wasn't the purpose of these diets—unless you do actually intend to start eating their strange meals permanently. As a result, by adopting a fad diet, you undertake two separate challenges: a diet to lose weight and a diet to maintain your new weight. Unless you follow up the first challenge by adopting and continuing the second challenge—which most often dieters fail to do—the weight will come right back.

A few years ago (seventeen, in fact, by the date of this writing), Jared Fogel, a 425 pound college student, embarked on a diet of two Subway® sandwiches every day as lunch and supper, a strategy that enabled him to lose 200 pounds and gain a career in public relations for Subway. His plan worked for him, and apparently he did learn how to keep the weight down. However, his strategy would hardly work for most people, and it fits nicely into the category of a fad diet. Don't try this at home.

Another fad diet is the Atkins Diet,™ a low carbohydrate strategy. Atkins qualifies for fad status because it requires the nearly complete elimination of carbohydrates from daily intake. Bread, rice, potatoes, crackers, sugar, and just about anything else that is vaguely white get the boot, while meat and lots of leafy or watery vegetables dominate your meals. If you don't already like pork rinds, get some and get used to them, because they become your new snack.

The diet induces a bodily response called ketosis, which is the conversion of stored body fat to energy. The byproducts of this conversion are expelled in more frequent urine. You literally pee away pounds; thus, you lose weight. After a while on the first stage of the diet, called Induction, Atkins switches to (OWL) Ongoing Weight Loss, then Pre-Maintenance, and finally Lifetime Maintenance, all of which depend on your going by prescribed foods and require you to avoid eating one thing while upping your intake of another.

The problem with Atkins or other versions of the low

carb strategy is that even after you near or achieve your target weight, you continue to have to consult lists of foods, until or unless you memorize them, and you wind up still paying a lot of attention to the diet. You may also find that your food restrictions determine whether or not you can even go out to eat at a particular restaurant, because its offerings may all be verboten, unless they serve simple rabbit food.

3. Diet Pills

Not as popular as they once were, diet pills or other preparations marketed either to depress appetite or increase metabolism are hailed as an easy way to lose weight—just pop a pill and the part with the pounds. Part of the reason pills are not as popular nowadays is that many of the drugs that emerged as diet aids have been disapproved by the FDA, including ephedra and phenylpropanolamine. Companies keep coming up with new chemicals they claim will boost metabolism, block fat, or stimulate the thyroid, but often sparse clinical studies support the claims, or if there are studies they show the drugs to be only marginally effective. Of late, more herbal aids then ever have emerged as dietary wonders, and almost never are they accompanied by scientifically conducted studies confirming their makers' boasts.

The problems with diet pills are several: not only do they often not work, but even when they do, they may have bothersome side effects. In addition, of course, the pills themselves are usually expensive: dieters are often desperate, and desperate people often spend more money than they should for vacuous promises.

Of course, the problem with pills is still the same as with other diet solutions that don't stress the discipline of the dieter. When the target weight is reached and the pills are discontinued, whatever suppression of appetite or artificial increase in metabolism or blockage of fat they may have provided, is discontinued along with them, and the dieter stands an excellent chance of regaining her weight promptly. The pill was essentially the only reason the weight came off, and when the pill is gone, the weight will return.

4. Supplied Food

Supplied Food diets are plans utilizing the services of companies that ship you the food you eat on your diet. Nutrisystem® is perhaps the best known of these services. Other products include Medifast®, Jenny Craig®, Weight Watchers®, etc. If you don't stray from what the food supplier sends, you *will* lose weight, because the meals and snacks are carefully designed to provide a tightly controlled number of calories that is less than what you would need to maintain your body fat.

What happens when you reach your goal? It depends. Have you learned to cook the way they do? No. Are you willing to weigh everything, consult tables of ounces and calories, and figure out how to create low calorie sauces? Probably not. Do you even know what substitutes were used for the real thing in their various concoctions? Almost certainly you don't. So, when the food regimen is over, the weight will come back unless you have already learned, or very quickly *do* learn, to prepare the type and amount of food that will enable you to keep the weight off. Having your own chef, if only a very remote one, may be exactly what you need, but of course, it comes at a price, and a fairly hefty one at that. Nutrisystem® works, but you have to do something other than eat their food. You have to learn another discipline separately in order to succeed long term.

The Point

It's pretty obvious that the most successful method of losing weight is the one that addresses the fundamental reason you gained weight in the first place. It cannot be stated more simply than this: you ate more food than your body needed. This is the definition of overeating. Getting rid of the unwanted weight is just as simple: eat less food than your body needs to maintain its fat. *Undereat.*

When I say "simple," I don't mean that it will be easy to undereat; I mean only that there is no mystery to it, no complex theory to understand about it, and no difficult strategy to adopt to accomplish it. It's simple: eat less.

To be most successful, you need to lose weight through a method that *by its very nature* creates a new sort of habit: self control. You need to learn how much food your body needs to maintain your target weight, and to be satisfied with that amount of food.

If part of that process means learning to eat a better balance of foods, add that discipline to your overall weight loss plan. Some people eat far more meat then they need, compared to vegetables. Conversely, some people have shied away from meat because of the influence of vegetarians or vegans, or because they heard some pseudo doctor tell them they should stop eating meat. Because they've swallowed popular but mistaken advice, they're eating too little meat—their protein intake isn't sufficient to deal with their carbohydrate intake. A balance of protein and carbohydrate is ideal. However, the core of the successful plan is simply learning to eat *less* than you used to.

To accomplish the goal of eating less, unless at the present you are subsisting on donuts, candy and sodas, you probably do not need to eat something else, and you do not

---

Nobody needs to make money off you
for you to lose weight.

---

need to buy anybody's service or plan or calculator. You don't need anyone to ship you anything or medicate you with anything. You don't need to buy bottles of pills at a pharmacy or herbal center. Nobody needs to make money off you for you to lose weight. If you bought this book instead of borrowing it, you just paid the last money you ever need to spend on dieting. You don't need to become anyone's customer or devotee to lose weight. You just need to eat less of what you have always bought at the grocery store.

This is what I mean by, *It's Amounts; that's all!*

ARE YOU AN EXCEPTION?

Some people, particularly among those who are very sensitive about their weight, raise an objection to any diet recommendation. They claim they have some medical condition that makes them overweight. The usual culprit is a thyroid condition, such as what is popularly referred to as a thyroid imbalance. People who claim to have some glandular condition, or who simply claim they have an abnormally low metabolic rate (for unknown reasons) staunchly resist any admission that they overeat.

Among these defensive folks a very small number *may* be correct. "According to the American Association of Clinical Endocrinologists (AACE), 27 million Americans have thyroid disease, but more than half remain undiagnosed."[2] Even if we take that figure at face value, that means only about 13-14 million people have known thyroid issues, and only some of these will be found to be overweight because of those conditions.

Even among those few people who are overweight in part or whole because of a thyroid imbalance, some of them got that way by taking prescription drugs that interfere with the thyroid. A great many more of them, mostly women, got that way by failing to eat a balanced diet and, if necessary, taking vitamin supplements.

If you are one of those people and you know it for a

---

[2]Vicky Uhland, "The Hidden Epidemic: Is Your Thyroid Making You Fat?" *Alternative Medicine* (2015), *http://www.alternativemedicine.com/thyroid/ hidden-epidemic-your-thyroid-making-you-fat.*

medical fact, simply put down this book. It isn't for you. If you are still reading and it's because you've just been guessing that you had a thyroid imbalance, and if you have been blaming your excess weight on something beyond your control, but you're willing to admit you may have been making an excuse, that's a start. Since eating less won't harm you, read on, and give it a shot. Finally, if you're a person whose metabolic rate really is lower than it used to be—for instance, because you're over sixty instead of under thirty (sorry; we just have to admit it at some point, don't we?), then keep reading, because there is no way to raise your natural metabolic rate:[3] you simply must eat less, and that's what this book is all about.

So scrap all your fad diet books and throw away all the phone numbers you copied down during TV commercials about how to lose weight on some fantastic plan that someone somewhere has just discovered. Don't even follow this book for your diet, but rather be *inspired* by it. I won't give you a diet plan in the sense of any daily foods, calorie targets and the like. I give you a philosophy, motivation, inspiration, and challenge. The rest is up to you, and you *can* do this. Believe me. Believe in yourself.

---

[3]You can raise your metabolic rate temporarily by exercise. Your normal rate, however, will not change, apart from disease, except pharmacologically, for other medically prescribed indications.

3
It's Amounts
That's All

Where other approaches to dieting are beset with fundamental weaknesses, the obvious tactic of eating less has no fundamental weakness at all. If it did, then you would have to conclude that the act of eating itself is fundamentally flawed: such a notion is the wrong-headed and harmful concept behind anorexia, which I thoroughly reject. What I'm talking about is eating *less*, compared to

---

As a strategy for weight loss,
eating less is unassailable.

---

eating *more* than is required to maintain a healthy weight. Eating smaller *amounts* can be looked at as eating *just the right amount,* nothing more, and as a strategy for weight loss eating less is unassailable. It's *amounts:* that's all.

It's not that people always succeed using this simple approach; it's just that if you follow this approach with discipline, it *will* work and it will *not* result in any side effects or leave negative aftereffects.

In a way, I feel it should be unnecessary to write a book about what really is an obvious fact, that eating less results in weight loss. However, the popular culture has perpetrated the hoax that you can blame obesity: on evil corporations for their sinister creation of foods overloaded with empty calories that render you helplessly fat; on a plethora of common foods that are inherently bad for you; on unknown environmental influences that doom you to being overweight; or on some other bogeyman of genetics or American foods or Western society in general. This hoax has underwritten the creation of one diet business after another, which seek to convince us, by repetition and slick advertising, that without at least one of their products or services, we will be morbidly fat all our lives. Thanks to them, however, on their diets we can lose five pounds in the first week, *for free!* That's the claim.

What I want you to see is that you can lose those five pounds, and the five after that, and the ten after that, *all* for free, that in fact you don't have to spend a dime to lose weight. All you have to do is eat less, and nobody is going to charge you anything for the privilege.

So, I want you to stop counting calories, right now. You aren't going to need to. You're going to learn to judge the amount of food you need by the look of it on your plate and by the way you feel at mealtime and in between meals. You're going to relearn to eat what you need, when you need it, without doing anything more complicated than that. It's not about counting, or calories, or carbs or any other strategy that requires you to plan this or restrict that or leave out something or substitute anything else.

It's amounts. That's all. It's how much you eat. It can't get any simpler than that.

If there are rules to this diet of a*mounts,* the first one would be to eat *whatever* kind of food you like.

EAT WHATEVER YOU LIKE

Think about the logic of this method. First, what effect have previous diets had on you when they restricted your intake of sugar? You craved sugar. Even if you settled into your sugar-free diet until you lost a few pounds, when you got off the regimen, what did you want? Most likely, it was sugar. Same with fat. Same with carbohydrates.

Similarly, if you went on a diet that majored in low calorie solutions involving substitution of non-fat substances for cream, butter, and so on, what did you want after a few days? Cream, butter, whole milk, maybe bacon grease and other things as well.

The point is that denying yourself the substances you love simply sets up a craving for those substances. The craving is created by the denial.

Those of you familiar with the story of Adam and Eve in Eden, will remember that the only thing denied to the first couple was the fruit on the tree in the middle of the garden. The observation is often made that being denied that fruit made it all the more appealing. The story of Eden actually says that the Serpent tempted Eve with that very notion—false, but effective—that God had denied Adam and her that particular fruit because he knew if they ate it, they would know as much as he did. That story is where we get the term "forbidden fruit" referring to something you can't have, legitimately at least, but which you want intensely.

It's even worse when you *have had* something for a long time and suddenly are told you can't have it. In my case, I eat just about everything. I dislike very few foods. Raw oysters come to mind, and okra. You couldn't name five other foods I have had that I don't like. I love spinach. If you told me I couldn't have spinach on some sort of diet, I would say no to the diet. Same with Brussels sprouts; no one else in my family would choose them as among their dozen favorite vegetables, but I would.

Fortunately, no diet in the world, I think, would deny me spinach or Brussels sprouts. Unfortunately, most diets would tell me not to have cheesecake, and I absolutely love cheesecake. And créme brulét. And really rich ice cream. If you share these loves or something similar, the good news is that since "it's *amounts*, that's all," you can have these things you love.

The key is to eat them without going overboard. Just how do you do that? Let's take a few examples. You can come up with other examples and devise other strategies on your own.

Plan for Desserts
Planning for desserts means one of two things:

• You can work them into your meal plan. On the day you plan to have a rich dessert, eat a very small breakfast and a harmless lunch—for instance, a salad crammed with tasty vegetables and just enough dressing to moisten it. I mix mine in a serving bowl and slice up lettuce, several kinds of peppers, tomato, celery, onion (very important to liven up a salad), carrots (grated), and some parsley. Add anything else that looks interesting in the crisper drawer of the fridge. For this particular salad, don't include any meat or cheese. Then, if you planned to have spaghetti that night, and you'd really like to have cheesecake for dessert, minimize the bread you might eat with the spaghetti, eat a small, vegetable salad on the side, serve yourself a modest amount of spaghetti and sauce, and don't go back for seconds—that's important: remember, it's *amounts*. Drink a half glass or small glass of tea or other beverage. Then have dessert. Cut a narrow slice of cheesecake, but enjoy it without guilt. If you were to add up the calories—which you're not going to do, because it's *amounts,* that's all—you would find that even with the cheesecake you didn't overdo it.

• The other method of planning for desserts is to make a very rich dessert your entire meal, or nearly so.

Let's say I have a hankering for ice cream—such cravings hit me now and then with volcanic force. I've had breakfast, and my supper is likely to be meat and three. What should I do for lunch? I can eat ice cream, and nothing else. I could go home and eat a bowl there, but the ritual and ambiance of an ice cream shop are often part of the enjoyment. There's an ice cream store down the road that sells nothing but ice cream on one side and markets peaches on the other side. It has picnic tables outside under a shed, and lots of local folks go there to smell the peaches while they eat bowls and cones of ice cream fresh from the churn. I sometimes go there for a medium cup as my whole meal. I get what I want but I don't mess up my diet.

Those of you who have been convinced by alarmist dieticians that at any given time you are only twenty-four hours away from serious nutritional imbalance, please sit down and calm yourselves. Eating dessert as your entire meal now and then will not threaten your health. I won't

---

The average person gets enough vitamins and minerals without thinking about it.

---

attempt in this book to go into the side issue of nutrition, but you can rest assured that the average person gets enough of the famous Recommended Daily Allowance (RDA) of food types and vitamins and minerals, without even thinking about it and without calculating or weighing anything. Since you're not going to eat dessert three meals a day, you're obviously going to get those veggies and fruits at another meal. Stop worrying.

Pick a smaller plate

If you're like our family, you have several sets of dishes. The first set we purchased (or were given) when we got married. It has dinner plates but no smaller, "lunch" size plates. Of course, we have formal dinnerware, and we use it so infrequently that I really think we should sell it, but my wife brings it out at Christmas, Easter and Thanksgiving, with a great sense of celebration and ritual. We also have a second set of daily "china," and it has two plate sizes. One is 11" in diameter, the other only 9".

Pick a 9" plate. If you don't have one, go to Goodwill and find a couple, one for you and one for your significant other, especially if he/she is also trying to lose weight. For dinner, get out these smaller plates, and when you spoon up your meat and three, the plate will invite you to serve smaller portions. Don't crowd the plate, and don't ever, ever make two layers of anything.

I watch people at the local Chinese buffet I frequent as they come from the steam tables, their plates stacked with three layers and then a Pike's Peak of fried shrimp on top of the whole thing. I think to myself, Don't they know they can go back? In fact, they do know that, and they plan to. And that, more than anything in the world, explains their weighing 350lbs.

That smaller plate will be a badge of pride for you. You will "fill" it—not cram it, just gently fill it—and you will enjoy it, and because you will not go back for more, whether you're at home or at a buffet, you will not overeat for that meal.

Allow yourself the occasional buffet

Since I've mentioned buffets, I'll go ahead and say what

most diet gurus naysay: allow yourself the occasional buffet. Your strategy is *amounts,* remember? You aren't going to go to a buffet every day; that question is answered by applying the *amounts* principle to the issue of buffets in the first place. You are, however, going to allow yourself to eat at a buffet now and then. What you're going to do is simply to treat the availability of food on the buffet the same way you would treat the presence of food in your refrigerator or on your stove top: you're going to take only what you need to sustain you and nothing more.

Two of my favorite places to eat are buffets: Ryan's (an American food spread), and New China (obviously, Oriental food). Recently I had planned to eat a salad for lunch at home by myself, but I needed to have a working lunch with a coworker. I suggested to him that we go to New China (he loves it, too). We both had water with lemon, and we both made one and only one trip to the buffet. Since we were talking a lot, we were busy with our mouths doing that, and since we picked the things we really liked from the buffet, we were satisfied with what we got the first time around. The result was a sensible meal.

Now, let me address some things you probably thought about when you read the previous paragraph.

• First, you probably thought about the general prohibition prominently preached by diet experts: No more buffets! They say this to you because they assume you are a person without discipline who will do what all those truly immense people do who build little volcanos of food on their plates and then go back again and again, and then have dessert.

The gurus *assume* that you cannot control yourself, and they want you to deny yourself the pleasure of some really good food at some of those wonderful restaurants. I sometimes think that diet gurus are sadists who want you to feel deprived.

I want you to feel at liberty to eat what you want. If that means Chinese food, and you can't cook Chinese food worth anything, and the Chinese restaurants nearby are all buffets, you are at liberty to go to one. Remember, *it's amounts, that's all!* You're going to go, pick four or five things you really like, take portions that add up to what you really need to sustain your energy and nothing more, and you're not going to go back for more. And you can skip desserts, because hardly any Chinese restaurant anywhere has really good desserts. They always look interesting, but they're almost always disappointing.

My wife and I occasionally go to a buffet and we take note of the many rotund people there. She used to turn to me and say We shouldn't come here anymore. But we do go back, because the food is very good and sometimes neither of us feels like cooking. However, we have developed the ability to eat only as much as we need, or even less. Seeing the sad results of indulgence apparently has served mostly as a disincentive to our following suit.

• The second thing you probably thought of was the idea that restaurant food is all loaded with fat or sugar or salt or something else you've been told is bad for you. Doubtless you can find restaurants whose offerings are heavy on grease or something else. For that matter, some things you cook at home will be fatty. However, you need to lay aside the idea that these foods are *bad* for you. I know: you think it's sacrilege to discard what the food police have told you all your life, but for the most part, you can.

Think of the number of times some authority—self-proclaimed, quasi or even bonafide—has told you that something is bad for you, only for you to find out years down the road that it really isn't. Coffee comes to mind. Caffeine has been condemned for years by this or that expert, but recently equally knowledgeable experts have confirmed what I always knew in my heart, that caffeine is not only not inherently bad for you, it can be very beneficial. In fact, although you've heard for years that caffeine is bad for your heart, recent discoveries show that regular caffeine intake actually helps regulate heart rate, and that coffee has no significant negative effects on almost anybody. As with most things that are part of our daily diets, *it's amounts* that make the difference.

Or take butter. Bad, right? No, in fact, recent and very high quality research has informed the waiting world that butter is just fine, thank you. In February 2015 various reports showed that the nervous trend of producers and consumers to switch from whole milk, real butter and substitutes for cream, which traces to 1983, was based on research that even at the time was flawed, being based on a study that consisted of materially conflicting results looking at a very small group of unhealthy men. Newer reviews of the growing body of evidence suggest strongly that "there is no association between heart disease and those fats."[4]

In respect of butter, compared to some of the substitutes, it's a whole lot better. The issues boil down to tradeoffs and the possible effects of the additives in artificial substitutes. For my part, I've been eating real butter for years. When I got married, I told my wife that we would have real butter on our table from day one. She could use margarine if she wanted (and she rarely wants to), but I was having butter. I have now been vindicated.

Or take salt. If you slavishly follow the experts (mostly those who get paid to enslave you) you go hunting for things on the supermarket aisles that say "low sodium." To be accurate, they should be talking about actual salt, not sodium. Salt is sodium chloride, but nothing you buy *ever* has just sodium in it. And since sodium is a element in many other chemical compounds in our environment, including our food, we should be measuring the content of salt, not sodium per se.

All that aside, you've heard the frantic advice and warning: Salt is bad! Unfortunately, it's not true in any absolute way.

Granted there are a few medical conditions exacerbated by excessive salt, but salt is a necessary element in our bodies, and most people's bodies deal with salt just fine, thank you. In fact, the premise that salt leads to hypertension (high blood pressure) has never been scientifically

---

[4]Jenny Hope, "Butter Isn't Bad for You After All," *Daily Mail* (June 1, 2015) *http://www.dailymail.co.uk/health/article-2946617/Butter-ISN-T-bad-Major-study-says-80s-advice-dairy-fats-flawed.html,* Accessed June 1, 2015.

supported.[5] I'll bet you didn't know that. Even some doctors have just accepted the common wisdom, which turned out to be the common fallacy, that salt is bad. Doctors can be wrong, too. They know what they study and then continue to read, and if the prevailing wisdom of a few people who write the books and disseminate the studies and reports are wrong about their research and conclusions—as they were about salt—then every doctor who just goes by what he reads in the medical journals is going to pass along to the rest of us the faulty advice.

The premise that salt leads to high blood pressure has never been scientifically supported.

In the case of salt, the American Journal of Medicine finally reversed itself and reported that people with reduced salt diets had significantly higher mortality rates than those who didn't deny themselves salt. We've also discovered that salt improves insulin sensitivity which helps control excess blood sugar; so a healthy dose of salt works against diabetes. There are at least eight other ways that salt is vital to body functions where too little salt will most certainly hurt, not help you.

---

[5] Note for example the comments of Dr. Malcolm Kendrick: "One of the most pervasive and stupid things that we are currently told to do is to reduce salt intake. This advice has never been based on controlled clinical studies, ever. Yet, as with the cholesterol myth, the dogma that we should all reduce salt intake has become impervious to facts." — Malcolm Kendrick, *Salt is Good for you, http://drmalcolmkendrick.org/2014/05/13/salt-is-good-for-you,* Accessed May 29, 2015.

This matter of salt comes into the discussion when the critics of buffets wag their fingers at us. Buffets in particular are commonly accused of being heavy on the salt. I don't let it worry me. I don't add any salt to buffet foods, anyway, and after all, I'm not going to eat there three meals a day, or probably not even three times a week. It's just not something I need to get myself into a tizzy about—or you, either. As it turns out, we need salt.

It's a good thing, too, because while I don't just pick up the salt shaker for everything on my plate at home either, I don't leave it out of anything that needs it, and I don't use salt substitute. Please join me in simply rejecting the idea that you need to be scared of regular foods and seasonings. There are killjoys in government, in alarmist organizations, and among your friends and neighbors, who are deathly afraid that eating normally spells disaster. It may be the exact opposite.

• A third thing you may have thought of as an objection to the so-called sage advice about avoiding buffets is that if you skimp when you go there, you'll waste money. My wife is inclined to think this way, but then, she won't buy staples we're out of because they don't happen to be on sale that particular week. There's such a thing as taking frugality too far. (I cut her some slack, however, because she makes up for it in many other, wonderful ways!)

Think about this for a minute. One of my local Chinese restaurants that is *not* a buffet serves a lunch special of Mandarin Chicken for $8.50, that comes with fried rice and egg roll. The Chinese buffet I frequent charges $6.99 for its lunch buffet. Even if I get the same foods, and only one extra egg roll or spring roll on the buffet, I've gotten the same food for the even less at the buffet, even without going back for seconds. I could compare typical meat & three places with my favorite all-American food buffet, and I would come up with similar results. I could try hard to find an inequitable pairing, but what would that prove? Nothing.

The point is that just because you *can* go back at a buffet doesn't mean you have to, either to stuff yourself or just to feel that you've gotten your money's worth.

So, eat whatever you want. That generalization applies

Just because you can go back at a buffet doesn't mean you have to.

---

whether your eating at home or eating out. Eating whatever you like therefore means:

EAT WHEREVER YOU LIKE

Do you like steak at fancy steak restaurants? Go. Go without hesitation. In fact, you may be able to eat less even easier at very fancy restaurants because of their penchant for putting small portions in the middle of large plates and drizzling some flambé-ed concoction over it in decorative squiggles. The dollop of potatoes wouldn't sustain an infant, much less you. If you don't bite for the tempting triple chocolate decadence they offer as a fantastically overpriced dessert, you'll actually go home wanting a snack long before bed. You can resist that temptation, too, because you will have succeeded in undereating for supper and you will be able to congratulate yourself that your resistance to indulgence will have already resulted in a few ounces weight loss, in addition to whatever you achieved through minimizing breakfast and lunch.

Eat pizza. Go to the parlor, order a medium meat extravaganza pizza for two, eat two pieces, no more, and slowly at that, while you talk a lot and have fun. Have the waiter put the other half of the pie in a box, then carry it home and put it in the freezer, where you will extract it next Sunday night and heat it up one piece at a time for a lazy supper while watching a ball game in the den. This also works for carry-out, of course. At this writing, only last night my wife and I ordered a medium pepperoni and Italian sausage pizza (not large, as we used to do) and picked it up fifteen minutes later. We each ate two pieces and froze the other half of the pie. In either case, the pizza cost about $10.00, but you and your significant other, if you have one, will get two meals out of it, so it will cost you $5.00, or $2.50 apiece. Not bad, I'd say.

Go to the Italian restaurant. Olive Garden is popular. Just remember, *it's amounts* that count, not ingredients. The ever popular Chicken Parmesan at Olive Garden is scrumptious, and it's made with lots of heavy cream. Don't be scared of it: just minimize your intake. Again, the technique of carrying half your dinner home in a take-out box is a wildly successful way of controlling the amounts you eat, and it halves your cost of the meal, since you get another whole meal out of it. Sometimes my wife and I will actually cut the food on the plate down the middle, and ask for the take-out box first. That helps insure we don't "accidentally" eat three fourths of the meal before "remembering" we were going to take the rest home.

Go out for breakfast. IHOP is popular, as is Cracker Barrel. Both restaurants offer smaller portion meals, if you want to go that way, or you can still eat half, or two thirds, and take the rest home for a light lunch or another breakfast.

Go to fast food restaurants. No, seriously. Your strategy there will be to share. I love the Burger King Whopper® and I don't care what its critics have to say about it. If I denied myself the occasional Whopper® I would revolt against the diet that constrained me to do so. The trick is eating only part of it. Since fast food burgers are not very good saved for another meal, even the very next one, plan to eat the Whopper® when there are two of you going. Cut it in half. That goes for the fries if you get them. Drink water to minimize the impact of even the half burger you do eat, or split a cup of tea. Voila. You've just made a diet-worthy meal of what most people think would blow any diet they might be on.

Remember: it's not where you go to eat: *it's amounts, amounts, amounts!*

EAT EVERYTHING YOU EAT SLOWLY

Somewhere in the dim and misty recesses of the past, when I was a little lad frequently visiting my paternal grandfather's house during the 1950s, he gave this sage advice, his being an octogenarian: eat slowly. Chew your food longer.

This is ubiquitously common advice; it can be found as a rule for almost every diet plan. Everyone from your local doctor to WebMD to the National Institutes of Health to experts on Zen (if you're into that, which I'm not) recommends eating slowly. Chewing thoroughly allows saliva to jumpstart the digestion process. Taking time between bites instead of stuffing down food rapidly allows the biochemical triggers of satiety (being full) to tell your brain you can stop eating. Eating slowly also often fills up the time you have to eat a meal, such as when you're on a lunch break. Multiple reasons exist to eat more slowly than you probably do now. For purposes of this book, the most important one is that if you eat slower, you will eat less, and that's our goal: *it's amounts!*

So, eating more than you needed got you where you are, and eating less than you need will get you back. Staying on the road to slim means exercising the discipline you already have to eat less, until you arrive at your goal. Instead of doing something strange or giving someone else your money for their promises, you are going to eat whatever kind of food you want, wherever you choose to eat it, enjoying it slowly.

But what about the inconsistency and failures you expect to encounter? Let's deal with those issues now.

4
Dealing with Detours
Getting Back on the Road

Y ou can readily imagine that the ideal diet would consist of a daily routine of eating that chopped off enough calories to amount to a pound or two per week of weight loss. Some people would want to make faster progress than that, but medical experts agree that losing much more weight than that in a week is unhealthy for numerous reasons. Without going into detail, such severe weight loss can upset body chemistry, temporarily reduce your metabolism (a bodily defense against starvation, which is counterproductive to your dietary goals), result in constipation, and lead to urinary problems including kidney stones. The side effects of excessively rapid weight loss are not worth it.

Pacing yourself at a rate of a couple of pounds per week involves consistent undereating—the reverse of your previous pattern of overeating—which in theory should be easy to accomplish, and most of the time it really is. One of the problems you will face, however, is the inconsistency between days when you are on a roll and find it relatively easy to eat less, and that day or two here and there when you have the seemingly uncontrollable urge to stuff yourself with high calorie foods of any and all kinds. Or, you manage to behave yourself at the table but when you're alone you get into a stash of candy or snacks and undo any progress you have been making. We're talking about cravings.

MANAGING CRAVINGS

Cravings are natural and you may expect them to take place periodically. They are little detours on your road to thin by controlling amounts. But how do you deal with these detours? I'm not going to go into great detail here; most of the solutions are glaringly simple.

First, you need to recognize the difference between a

Cravings are natural...
expect them to take place periodically.

---

psychological rebellion against your imposition of a diet on yourself, on the one hand, and on the other hand, a physio-logical demand by your body for calories to burn instead of drawing on fat reserves. In other words, sometimes you're just tired of the diet, but sometimes your body really does need an infusion of quickly metabolized energy. The craving may seem the same, but while you can probably talk yourself out of the psychological urge to break with your diet, you will find it nearly impossible to quell the jittery urgency of a physiological craving. Plus, the physiological urgency often will center on a particular kind of food: carbohydrates, for instance. That's one way to tell the difference between the two kinds of cravings.

Occasionally, however, the two cravings may be combined. I experienced one of these combination cravings during one year many moons ago, when I underwent significant weight loss. I remember a day when I had the intense desire to eat candy. It was around Christmastime, and there were cans, jars and dishes of candy in nearly every room. The day before the craving began, the visibility of candy wasn't a problem, but then suddenly it was. I've always loved candy, and I wanted candy; it was as simple as that. And there it was. I ate hard candy, filled candy, chocolate peppermint bark, and sweet coated nuts. There were expensive chocolates in a box in the pantry, and I ate those (not all of them). There were cookies in a drawer that I had ignored for a month, but that day, I raided them. I knew I was blowing it, but I didn't care. I had been good, very good, during a season you celebrate in part by eating big meals and sweet treats, and I felt denied by keeping myself away from them. Not only was I undereating and forcing my body to raid its fat supplies for energy, but I was doing so while surrounded by visual cues as to how rapid energy— sugar—could be found. That day, my continuing self-deprivation intersected overwhelming temptation and I succumbed. It ended only when I went to bed.

The next day, I calmly returned to my controlled diet. I looked at the candy dishes and jars, didn't move them from their decorative places, and didn't want any of what was in them. I had no problem saying No. The craving was gone. It didn't return the next day or the next, either.

Dealing with the psychological war can be difficult; there's no point in leading you to believe otherwise. You can try hypnosis, and some people have, but outside of paying someone to put you under hypnosis very deeply—the kind of a trance that you don't remember—the results of the fully-awake sort of hypnosis are minimal at best. You can join a support group of some kind, such as Overeater's Anony-mous, and support groups are not a bad idea, anyway; but group or no group, *you* make the final decision about whether or not you're going to eat something, or how much of it. At its core, the battle is going to be won only by personal commitment. Will power. Discipline. There are no substitutes for this commitment. Return to Chapter 1 and review the discussion of this subject if you need to.

DEVELOPING COMMITMENT

So, how do you develop the commitment? For some people, this development isn't as hard as it is for others; they make a decision and stick with it. They exercise what I called earlier the innate capacity for discipline. Why they didn't decide to stay slim in the first place could be for many reasons, but finding themselves needing to lose weight, they take their innate ability, flex their disciplinary muscles and hold fast to their decisions. Other people have a lifelong war with their own wills; they have great difficulty keeping commitments.

For those who have trouble with willpower, the best remedy is practice. The best place to start is the actual field of battle: your diet. Start by choosing a meal at random, say, supper on Wednesday. For that meal, no matter where it is, at home or out, undereat significantly. Take less from serving bowls, order the smallest thing on the menu, and then eat only two thirds of what you have on your plate. If you drink a sweetened drink, say no to anymore than half of it. If you fail to follow through with undereating at this meal, pick another meal and try again.

When you have mastered limiting yourself at one meal, try the same technique for a day. Take one day at random, set a plan for cutting back by planning all three meals (don't skip any), and stick with that plan, knowing that tomorrow, you won't be doing it again. If you don't keep your promise to yourself, pick another day the next week and try again. Do that several weeks in a row. You are strengthening your ability to say no to overeating.

For a third, more prolonged "will-power workout," set aside a whole week to exercise your discipline. Count down the days, if you must, but stick to it for one week. If you blow it after two or three days, quit trying for the whole week, skip a week, and try again. When you can make it for a week eating, say, 2,000 or less calories per day, you have strengthened your ability to commit to a more significant diet. In the process, you will have lost two or three pounds while doing your "exercises."

In addition to practicing your sense of discipline in the area of eating, you will reinforce this training by getting some discipline into other areas of your life as well.

LEARNING FROM YOURSELF

If you are one of those people who have difficulty sticking with things, it is likely that you don't have this problem in absolutely every area of your life. Probably there are some things that you never thought twice about doing regularly with commitment, because you already find yourself sticking to those things faithfully. What are those things? Identify them and analyze what it is about those things that makes it easy for you to do them with devotion. This will help you address difficulties with your diet, as well as with other areas where commitment is spotty or lacking entirely.

For instance, if you have a job, do you get up at a certain time regularly, arrive at work on time, and have a routine at work that you keep rigorously? Why? Likely reasons will be that you won't get paid or might get fired if you don't do these things. On the positive side, you may be motivated by the constant awareness that you are accomplishing something in your job and you like the feeling it gives you to produce work that is of high quality or is praiseworthy. Is there anything about your motivations that might apply to losing weight?

Obviously, you aren't getting paid to lose weight. Or are

you? Aside from the blunt reality that some people are passed over for job promotions because of issues with their weight, there are other ways that losing weight pays you. A friend of mine whom I hadn't seen in about six months explained his very evident weight loss. He had been a diabetic for years, controlling the condition with oral medication. On a trip to the doctor, he was informed that henceforth he would need to take insulin by injection. He bargained with the M.D. and went on a diet. In six months

---

Every pound you lose
is equivalent to more horsepower.

---

he lost forty pounds, and was continuing downward. The diabetes was dramatically improved and he escaped having to start giving himself shots every day. Not only that, but he was also able to stop taking the oral medication. His weight loss paid him in real dollars.

I ride a motorcycle. It's a small cruiser, and from time to time I observed to my riding buddy that I wished the bike had more power. He tactfully said, "You realize that every pound you lose is equivalent to more horsepower." I added that prospect of reward to my bucket of the advantages of losing weight. It's tangible payback—whether you ride or not.

In what other activities or circumstances are you able to keep commitments? Are you married? Are you faithful? If you're married and you cheat now and then, you can skip this paragraph! Otherwise, note what it takes to keep your wedding vows. They're serious. They're made in a serious context. They are meant to be permanent. You think these things through before you make that kind of promise, and when you say, "I do," you mean it. Further, you are aware of both the future rewards and the prospect of negative consequences if you don't keep your vows. Mostly, however, you're thinking of what a wonderful thing it will be to be married. You don't think to yourself every day, "I might be miserable." You think instead, "This is going to be great!"

Apply these principles to losing weight. First, make a solemn commitment to yourself. Then rehearse the kind of attitude you're going to adopt for your challenge. Don't simply *avoid* thinking, "I'm going to hate this:" *start* thinking, "I'm going to really enjoy being lighter!" You're going to fit into smaller, more attractive clothes, perhaps some in the back of your closet or the bottoms of your chest of drawers. You're going to be able to shop at regular stores instead of the Big & Tall or the Stout Shop.[6] You're going to walk faster, get up more easily, stay active during the day longer, fit into chairs better, be more confident of your profile in public, be more attractive to your significant other or to a prospective one(!), and you're going to feel better all around. Make a list of things that are going to be great about losing weight!

---

[6]The well-known Catherine's Stout Shoppe renamed itself just Catherine's when "stout" and dozens of other words for being overweight became politically incorrect. If it walks like a duck…

Utilizing a Make-up Fast

What if, during the course of your diet, you simply lose the fight against a craving and give in "big time?" Let's say that on a Sunday you have a big dinner with the family, take seconds on everything because it tastes *so-o-o* good, and when you realize you've blown it, you figure, what the heck. You have desert, too—not just a piece of pie, but an extra wide piece. Knowing the day is shot, you eat a full supper as well, an extra thick hamburger, fries, and a 16-oz Coke. The modest breakfast you started out with was empty symbolism, as you have probably gained a whole pound during the day's eating, especially since you sat on the sofa between episodes of stuffing yourself, and you watched ball games. What now?

Consider a make-up fast, preferably the next day. Drink lots of water, adding lime or lemon juice if you like, but eat nothing the whole day. Don't tell yourself you can't do it, because you can. It's just one day. If you get a headache, as some people do from not eating, take whatever OTC NSAIDs you need (Non-Steroidal Anti-Inflammatory Drugs), such as acetyl salicylic acid, naproxin sodium, or ibuprofen (aspirin, Aleve, Tylenol, or Advil), drink plenty of water, and just tough it out for one day. In all likelihood, you couldn't have eaten enough the previous day to equal two days' calories, and a one day fast will make up for your indulgence and then some.

Mind you, this is *not* ideal. The plan is to undereat

consistently, not to indulge and then fast. There's little difference in the latter from binging and purging, which would be descriptive of a wholly different problem, bulimia nervosa. What you're after is training yourself to be regularly disciplined. Don't make a habit of fasting to make up for stuffing. In other words, don't say to yourself, I'm going to blow the diet big time next Sunday and then fast Monday. However, keep the possibility of a fast in your dietary arsenal to use when necessary.

Starving yourself for a whole day arguably takes more discipline than limiting yourself at three meals. As I say, however, this can be argued, and some would argue the reverse. Mark Twain, an avid cigar smoker, told how he was once advised by his doctor to moderate his habit, and he

---

Keep the possibility of a fast
in your dietary arsenal.

---

replied that he couldn't do it. He said he could quit entirely, but he couldn't moderate it. Some people would contend the same thing in response to the idea that they must be regularly disciplined. They'd rather fast a day here and there to make up for overeating than to contain themselves consistently. They think they would be unable to keep themselves from binges.

If that's your case, then you need to seek some counseling about addictive behavior, not just about food but about things in general. If you can't look at food and "just say no" when you need to, you have a problem that goes beyond an addiction to food. Nor is the answer simply to follow a different kind of diet that allows you to eat larger quantities; that very choice probably functions as an accommodation of addictive behavior. If that's the kind of tactic you regularly opt for, your life probably displays some glaring, dysfunctional lack of discipline in various areas.

EXPECTING DETOURS

On any journey of substantial length, you can expect some detours. Traveling your road to losing the excess weight you've accumulated is no different. Things will go perfectly some days and then you'll run into detours—those circumstances in which it's difficult to stick to the plan of eating less, or days on which you've simply veered off, following your appetite instead of your commitment.

For these times, imagine that you've got a dietary cell-phone road map with you all the time, programmed with that destination of being slender. A few minutes after you go off road by indulging in an unnecessary snack or you make a return trip to the buffet when you're really already full, your cell phone says, "Recalculating. Drive 300 feet then turn Right!" (I like mine to speak to me in a British accent—it seems more persuasive.) In this case, imagine her saying, "Recalculating. Walk to the next table and Leave the Buffet!" or "Return home and Eat Less!" When you take little detours on your diet trip, just recalculate, figure out a short route to get you back to where you were and put you back on track.

We've identified the strategy of undereating as the key to not only successfully losing the excess but also staying lighter for good. Now let's look at the internal, the essential, the spiritual core of dieting. Let's look at the *Thin Commandments* themselves.

5
The Thin Commandments
Principles for Getting and Staying Thin

To best understand the concept of the Thin Commandments, it's necessary to understand the context of the original Ten Commandments, the ones given to Moses in the Bible. To do that, first I'll give a little history lesson.

The family of Abraham moved into what was at the time Canaan. They proliferated there for three generations and then, in a time of great famine, they sought food from Egypt, where a wise CFO for the Pharaoh had planned well for drought and famine and had plenty to sell. In fact, the CFO was Joseph, one of the great grandsons of Abraham, who had been sold into slavery by his brothers and had risen to power because of his surpassing discipline and wisdom. After a series of events Joseph revealed himself to his brothers and invited the family to pack their camels and move down to Egypt for the duration of the famine.

They wound up staying there 430 years. After the first generation died, "there arose up a new king over Egypt, which knew not Joseph" (Exodus 1:8), and the Egyptian

Pharaohs made the Hebrews, Abraham's descendants, into slaves. Many scholars today believe that the Hebrew slaves built some of the later Egyptian monuments.

At any rate, after more than 400 years, Moses was born, who eventually demanded that Pharaoh let the Hebrew people go. After a series of awesome events now known as the ten plagues, Pharaoh freed the Hebrews and Moses led them out into the desert toward Canaan.[7]

The multitudes of people in the desert of Sinai were about to become something other than Hebrews; they were about to be Israel, the nation and the people of God. The key event that transformed them into Israel (which was also the name of Jacob, the father of the twelve tribes that originally went into Egypt) was the giving of the Law, the Ten Commandments, and their agreeing to abide by that law and to be God's people. That Covenant, as it was called, was the turning point in their national life.

The Ten Commandments are basically divided between man's direct relationship with God and his direct relationship with his fellow man. That pretty much covers everything. The most important thing we do when confronted with the Commandments is to see how they must be applied to our lives. That's where the water meets the wheel and the rubber meets the road. The Ten Commandments make an interesting plaque in front of a church or (controversially) a courthouse, but if that's all that's done with them, they're

---

[7]Estimates of how many Hebrews left Egypt vary widely. The mean number is around 600,000, but the best, biblically supported number is about 600,000 *men*. A total of more than 2,000,000 is not impossible.

only symbolic. Once we start applying them, we realize the principles they teach are all-encompassing, and we find upon even closer inspection that they speak to every area of life.

Accordingly, the *Thin Commandments* are principles for getting and staying thin, derived from the original Ten Commandments. They are the principles of the original Ten, boiled down to their plainly worded essence as applied to this one area of life: eating. If you have difficulty with one of them or feel like arguing with one of them, stop and consider where your objection really should be lodged.

Some years ago, I attended a nationwide convention meeting where a noted preacher was giving the keynote sermon. As he was delivering a particularly powerful challenge, someone in the vast crowd who took issue with him called out from the darkened arena, saying something critical. The preacher didn't miss a beat. He pointed in the general direction of the heckler and said, "Don't argue with *me,* sir; argue with the Bible—and then repent!"

These *Thin Commandments* come from the Ten Commandments of the Bible. If you take issue with them, leave me out of it. Take your complaint up with the one who gave the original Ten. You can write me later and tell me how it went.

THE THIN COMMANDMENTS

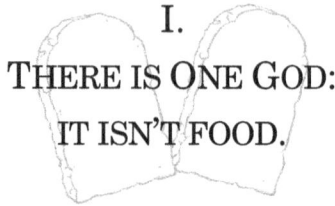

I.
THERE IS ONE GOD:
IT ISN'T FOOD.

The Original 1ˢᵗ Commandment:
I AM THE LORD THY GOD... THOU SHALT HAVE
NO OTHER GODS BEFORE ME (EXODUS 20:3).

The original first commandment made crystal clear that there is only one God—obviously there are other gods, with a little "g," because people worshiped all sorts of things, from elements of nature to sticks of wood and carvings of stone. However, there was and is only one God, the one greater than whom there is no other. That was the truth the Israelites were to start with. By the time of the New Testament, Jesus was teaching that people often served the god "Mammon," a term for money. Now, there's an up-to-date identification of the most common god of humanity.

A god is anything that is the most important thing in a person's life, the thing (or person) whom he serves, lives for, puts first in his efforts and use of time. To be certain, many people today live for money. Nothing is more important to them than making and amassing money. Running a close second to money is pleasure of all sorts. Often, what we spend our money for, especially out of proportion to the average person, will define a god.

Essentially, people can be polytheistic in this regard, because they serve several things that together are all-important to them—money, material possessions, sex, drugs, work, and—as you will realize if you think about it—food. Some people live to eat.

Even if we moderate that blunt assessment somewhat, we still have to admit that food is pretty high on the list of things to which some people give an inordinate amount of importance. Clearly, I don't mean that anything that's important is a god; that would indict the basics of shelter, clothing, food, health, and anything else that can be described legitimately as necessities. Even those things, however, can attain status as deities when they are elevated far above their necessity. Food qualifies as a god when it is much more important than it should be.

• When you value eating much more than being healthy, food is a god.

• When you value eating to the detriment of your family, food is a god.

• When you value eating to the point that it harms your relationships, your job, or your own bodily mobility, food is a god.

The 1st *Thin Commandment* is to get your priority right. If food is a god to you, take it off the throne of your life.

II.

FOOD IS TO BE EATEN,
NOT WORSHIPED.

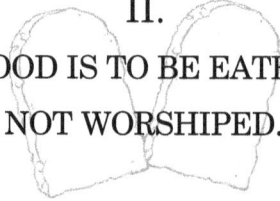

The Original 2ⁿᵈ Commandment:
THOU SHALT NOT MAKE UNTO THEE ANY GRAVEN IMAGE—
THOU SHALT NOT BOW DOWN THYSELF TO THEM,
NOR SERVE THEM (EXODUS 20:4-5).

The 1ˢᵗ Commandment proclaimed that YHWH (the English spelling of God's Hebrew name) was God—the only one. The 2ⁿᵈ Commandment followed up that basic fact with a logical and conclusory obligation: don't worship anyone or anything else. The tendency in ancient cultures was to make an image to represent a deity that people believed existed; think of the ancient Greek and Roman pantheons with dozens and dozens of major and minor deities, honored by statues of what sculptors thought these beings looked like. So the Hebrews, about to become the Israelites, were specifically told not to make visible idols to worship.[8]

The 2ⁿᵈ *Thin Commandment* is to treat food as what it is—something to be eaten for sustenance and enjoy-

---

[8]It's a mistake to think that the 2ⁿᵈ Commandment prohibited statues or other images altogether. The overwhelmingly clear force of the commandment is against worshiping such objects. "God is a Spirit, and they that worship him must worship him in spirit and in truth" (John 4:24).

ment—not to treat it as something it wasn't and isn't meant to be, virtually a god. I've already discussed how you can recognize whether food has godlike status to you. Perhaps you don't think you fit into the category of people who see food that way. What the 2nd *Thin Commandment* does is follow up with a prohibition of the activity or attitude that reveals what position food really takes in our lives.

What is worship?

Worship can be defined as showing reverence and adoration for, or honoring with extravagant love. I won't go to an unjustified extreme of suggesting to you that you should never say, "I *love* steak!" or "This pizza is to *die for!*" We don't really mean the latter, and in the former, we use the word "love" loosely quite often. What the 2nd *Thin Commandment* warns us against is living in such a way that we do, in fact, honor food above everything or even most things, or that we do, in fact, choose food over things (and people) that are much, much more important, or should be.

• Don't be ruled by food. You don't have to clean your plate if you don't want to.

• Don't obey food; it has a way of calling to us, doesn't it? Which is more powerful, you or the food?

• Don't give up other important things in your life because you eat too much. That sport or even mild activity you can't participate in because of your weight, is likely more important than your devotion to food.

- Don't jeopardize your health or life span by indulging slavishly in food. If you have a significant other, children, grandchildren, or siblings—even parents—who want you around for a while, what does it say that you may be cutting time off your life because you won't put down the fork?

A mess of pottage

Henry David Thoreau famously said, "I shall never thus sell my birthright for a mess of pottage,"[9] referring to overworking just to have things he might have wanted, but didn't need. The phrase, "a mess of pottage," refers to the Bible story about Jacob and Esau, though the exact words don't appear there. Jacob tricked a famished Esau into trading his birthright (his inheritance) for a bowl of pottage (stew). He was near home and wouldn't have starved, but he actually chose to take the mess of pottage in trade for his right to inherit from their father, Isaac, everything the firstborn would receive when Isaac died. What a bad deal!

"A mess of pottage is something immediately attractive but of little value taken foolishly and carelessly in exchange for something more distant and perhaps less tangible but immensely more valuable."[10] That immediate attraction certainly describes many a tantalizing meal or dessert, but it's not likely that you would be giving away your health or

---

[9]Henry David Thoreau, *Cape Cod, and Miscellanies, 460-461*; also *Life without Principle - 1*, 1863. *The Heart of Thoreau's Journals*, Odell Shepard, Ed., Dover Publications, Inc., New York 1961) 41.

[10]"Wickipedia, the Free Encyclopedia, *http://en.wikipedia.org/wiki/Mess_of_pottage#cite_note-16*, Accessed on 2 June 2015.

longevity by indulging in one meal, no matter how huge.

Months and years of overeating, however, are a different thing. For the immediate gratification, *day after day,* of stuffing ourselves far beyond our needs, we may well pay with the loss of our health and even the loss of our lives years before we might otherwise die.

Wimpy, the Popeye cartoon character, often said, "For the price of a hamburger today, I will gladly repay you Tuesday." The person who has allowed food to become a god to himself or herself probably will repay far more than the price of a hamburger, down the line somewhere. That makes thinking seriously about the place of food in your life a vital matter today.

Getting rid of the idol

Once coming into a covenant with God based on the Ten Commandments, the ancient Israelites were expected to get rid of their idols. To follow the *Thin Commandments,* how would you go about getting rid of the idol of food?

Obviously, you can't stop eating altogether. Food is a necessity. You must simply define what makes your food a god, what makes the way you eat or think about food an act tantamount to worship, and simply determine to act differently beginning now.

Nor am I suggesting that fancy meals, which by their nature celebrate food itself, are equivalent to food-idolatry. A banquet consisting of foods rarely found or difficult to prepare, served with flair and constituting a feast for the eyes as well as the tongue, does not qualify as an idol. You could eat modestly at a banquet, enjoying the delicacies and out-of-the-ordinary tastes, without going overboard. And again, even if you happen to stuff yourself (hey, banquets like that don't happen for most of us very often!), it's not the occasional feast that constitutes making an idol of food; it's a pattern of eating that does. Thanksgiving is still safe to observe!

What makes food an idol is eating more than you need, on a continual basis. When you overeat routinely, you are serving food, instead of its merely being served to you! There is *one* God; it's *not* food.

III.

A BLESSING BEFORE GLUTTONY IS TAKING GOD'S NAME IN VAIN.

The Original 3rd Commandment:
THOU SHALT NOT TAKE THE NAME OF THE
LORD THY GOD IN VAIN (EXODUS 20:7).

The 3rd Commandment prohibited a person's irreverent and disrespectful reference to God. It enjoined more than cursing. "In vain" broadly means to misuse, to speak emptily, to use words deceitfully, maliciously or falsely. So when the Serpent said to Eve, "God knows that on the day you eat the fruit, you'll be like gods," he was twisting the truth and attributing it to God—taking God's name in vain. Profanity using a name of God is included in the 3rd Commandment's prohibition, but it's by no means the only way of violating it. The positive way of stating the Commandment is to say that out of the utmost reverence for God we should never use his name in connection with anything but truth or blessing.

The 3rd *Thin Commandment* simply says we shouldn't ask God to bless our food if we're planning on making pigs of ourselves.

Again, I remind you that I'm not talking about the

occasional feast as it fits into an otherwise healthy way of eating. I'm talking about a pattern of gluttony.

Obviously, the 3rd *Thin Commandment,* by referring to saying a blessing, applies to those of you who make a habit of praying, or reciting a memorized blessing, before you eat. Not everyone does.

Let me chase a rabbit. The before-meal blessing is an interesting ritual. It has precedent in Jewish cultural life, and as such it seems to have been practiced by Jesus (a Jew of the tribe of Judah), and there is some evidence that it was practiced by Christians regularly, not just before ceremonial meals. The blessing consists of one or both of two elements: a statement of thanks for the food we are about to eat; and a request for God to bless it, or to bless our eating of it, such that we will use the strength we get from it to live for him.

Nothing in the Bible ever commands that a blessing be "said" before a meal. (We should probably refer to the practice as "asking a blessing," since that's what the act implies.) Nevertheless, because of the example appearing now and then in the Bible, Christians include it as one of the overt acts of devotion to God.

For the blessing sayers among us, then, how consistent are you between belief and practice? If you pick up a biscuit while driving to work and eat it while in the car, do you stop in traffic to say a blessing first? If you sit down with friends for Mexican food and eat chips and salsa, do you give thanks first, or only when your order comes—if then? (Restaurants often lead to dispensing with the blessing.) If there's something wrong with eating without first saying a blessing, shouldn't we feel guilty about the chips and salsa, or the glass of tea or cup of coffee we may be served first and probably sip on without pausing to pray? A friend of mine who fits into this category humorously dismisses this observation, but he acknowledges I've made my point.

I'm being somewhat tongue in cheek in this digression, but what it all leads around to is this: saying a blessing or asking for God's blessing on our food is indicative of thankfulness. At this point, many more of you would be included in the audience of the 3rd *Thin Commandment,* because even among those who don't practice the recitation of a blessing or a prayer of thanks before meals, quite a few of you would profess to be thankful for your food. In view of the fact that more than 70% of Americans claim to be Christians, I think it's safe to say that the vast majority of Americans would say they're thankful to God for their food, even if they don't "say thanks" before they eat.

Even if you don't, but you would profess to be thankful to God for your food in general, how does that thanksgiving jibe with continual, gluttonous overeating? Do you see the disconnect— even hypocrisy? Out of the utmost reverence for God we should not claim to be thankful to him for something we have every intention of then abusing. It makes a mockery of our profession, and dishonors him as well.

IV.
REMEMBER THE SABBATH:
GIVE YOUR FORK A REST.

The Original 4ᵗʰ Commandment:
REMEMBER THE SABBATH DAY,
TO KEEP IT HOLY (EXODUS 20:8).

Everything we do in life is subject to the general philosophy echoed by Ecclesiastes 3:1, "To every thing there is a season..." The writer didn't include a lot of things in the list he then gave, which started out, "a time to be born and a time to die." He didn't include eating, but it's implied, as are sleeping, working, playing, talking, and everything else. There's a time to eat and a time to stop eating. The 3ʳᵈ *Thin Commandment* is about knowing when to stop.

When I first thought of this *Thin Commandment,* I chuckled to myself, but only halfway. The original 4ᵗʰ Commandment was about keeping a day of rest once a week. The observance marked the Israelites as God's covenant people. It was based first upon their history, which said that God created in six days and rested on the seventh. Thus the seventh day, which was and still is what we call Saturday, was to be a sabbath. The word means cessation or rest. The Israelites immediately came to use the day of rest for more focused and extensive worship, and since various other sabbaths figured into their larger system of sacrifice, the title of Sabbath for the seventh day came to represent worship as well as rest. Most Christians have their day of rest and worship on Sunday, and many of them refer to it as their sabbath.

The 4th *Thin Commandment* is a blunt way of saying we should all know when to say, No more. I've discovered a great sense of satisfaction in being able to lay down the fork and say, "I've had enough."

I was raised by parents who went through the Great Depression and learned to clean their plates, not wasting food. When I was a child in the 1950s, the "Clean Plate Club" was no joking matter. There were sometimes real consequences for failing to eat everything on your plate—no dessert (of course), no TV after supper, and no snack later just because you got hungry: it was your own fault because you didn't clean your plate. When I became an adult, I realized eventually that my unconscious compulsion for eating every last bite of food I was served traced directly to my childhood rearing. Going against that early-learned pattern was extremely difficult.

I found, however, that if I thought of the idea of leaving a few bites on my plate as a challenge rather than as a temptation (as if I were doing something wrong), then I could rise to the challenge and do it. I realized I was establishing a new habit by ending my meal before my food was gone, and that it was one that would pay off in the short term as well as the long. In the short term, I wouldn't feel overfull when I left a restaurant; I would have quit before I got that far. In the long term, of course, I would eat less, and as I've said repeatedly in this book already, *it's amounts—that's all!* The most successful diet is all about simply eating less.

Giving your fork a rest is a challenge for the individual meal, and it's also a challenge for a daily meal plan.

- Plan to use your fork less in a single meal by taking smaller portions that won't take as many fork-fuls to eat.
- Put your fork down between bites; many diet plans advise this, and it works. It gives your stomach time to send the "all full" message to your brain.
- Leave a little food on the plate. Think of it as your concession to the ancient Arab custom: to them, eating every last bite implied an insult to your host, because it suggested he had given you too little.
- Take a portion of your meal home if you're eating out, or just put something in the fridge as a leftover if you're eating at home.

Giving your fork a rest is not meant to limit your life, but to free it and enable it. Eating less will make every meal more enjoyable. Stopping before you are uncomfortably full will keep you from regret and may prevent indigestion. The occasional fast, as I discussed earlier, has its own benefits.

To every thing there is a season: a time to eat and a time to refrain from eating. Learn when your sabbath from eating arrives, and give your fork a rest.

V.

HONOR YOUR PARENTS: THEY
WOULDN'T WANT YOU TO BE FAT.

The Original 5th Commandment:
HONOR THY FATHER AND THY MOTHER (EXODUS 20:12).

The 5th Commandment laid out God's expectation that in families, children should respect and obey their parents and not rebel against them. The family was and *is* the foundation of any society, and it could not be strong and resilient in an atmosphere where parents were dishonored.

The 5th *Thin Commandment* is simply a direct application of the original, in the narrow area of eating. Its restatement of the ancient law is couched in ideal terms, of course; the *ideal* parents would be fit and trim and would want their progeny to be fit and trim as well.[11] In fact, however, many people, and therefore many parents, are not fit and trim. *Some* of these parents care greatly about their children's physical condition and don't want them to be like their father and/or mother. Unfortunately, more often it's the case that fat parents have fat children. Go to Wal-Mart

---

[11]In reading this book this far, you realize that I'm not going to play the game some do, suggesting that there is no ideal because no body shape should be considered undesirable. It's one thing to decide to live with your weight and not try to change it, but quite another to pretend that obesity is beautiful.

to see examples.

I've heard some astounding rationalizations for this tubby-family tendency, including unsupported claims that they all have thyroid conditions or that fat runs in the family. Well of course it does. They all eat too much.

I'm very well aware that some geneticists believe there are genes that influence metabolism and appetite. One particular gene that's been identified is called FTO. About a fifth of the white population is believed to possess this gene, and people who have two copies of it in their DNA tend to weigh more. Researchers conclude that in people with this variant, the FTO gene "raises their risk of obesity."[12] But the doctor who led the study that made these findings said the gene "may be some kind of McDonald's gene or some kind of office chair gene."[13]

In other words, the key to this "birth gene," as FTO is being called, is that the findings show it isn't a problem in people born before 1942, and the only reason they can give for that curious fact is lifestyle—desk jobs, cars, and TV. The lifestyle of pre-WWII people differed radically. In any event, the researchers said the gene may be "activated" only under certain lifestyle conditions.

What does this tell you? It tells you rather loudly and forcefully that even *if* you happen to have some gene that gives you the *tendency* or the *possibility* of getting fat, it still

---

[12]Maggie Fox, "Will the 'Fat Gene' Get You? Your Birth Year May Matter," (NBC News, Dec 30, 2014) *http://www.nbcnews.com/health/health-news/will-fat-gene-get-you-your-birth-year-may-matter-n276366,* Accessed June 4, 2015.

[13]Dr. James Niels Rosenquist, commenting on the Framington Heart Study.

boils down to *how much you eat.*

Think about this rationally. No one has genes that make them fat if they don't eat at all. All of us have to eat something in order to keep living. If you have a gene that gives your body a bias toward becoming fat, that means mostly that you don't have to eat as much as the next person who is of the same height, age, and physical activity. It *doesn't* mean that no matter how little you eat, you'll still gain weight. It means only that to keep from gaining weight gradually, you must eat a little less than the next guy who doesn't have the genetic predisposition to weight gain. See that little phrase, "eat less," again? *It's amounts!*

For example, a male aged 50 years who is 6' 0" and is an office worker requires about 2,150 calories per day on average to sustain a weight of 185 lbs. The typical figure given for how many calories you have to skip in order to lose a pound is 3,500.[14] Of two men who could be described in this same way, one without the FTO genetic variant eats 2,150 calories per day and stays at 185 lbs. for five years. The other, who does have the variant, eats the same amount of food and does identical work, but he gains twenty pounds in five years. I'll spare you the math, but that works out to about a hundred calories per day the second man ate but didn't need to maintain his weight. That's a single piece of bread, or a large egg, a half cup of mashed potatoes, or a single ounce of steak.

---

[14]Recently, that figure has come under fire. It varies greatly with what kind of weight you lose and how you attempt to lose it. *Some* figure is going to be close, however. Averaging the various estimates at 3,500 is still useful.

Having a gene that gives you a tendency to gain weight *cannot* be blamed for your being overweight. When you have to get a bigger size in pants and belts, you know you're gaining weight and you know you could eat less and lose it. When you step on the scales and they say five pounds more than the last time you weighed a month ago, you know you could lose that weight by cutting back. You and I simply must be honest with ourselves that we cannot blame our weight on our parents.

That gets us back to the 5th *Thin Commandment*. What do our parents really wish we'd do about our weight?

Some of your parents are still with you, and a few of them have spoken to you about your weight. Overweight parents who have no room to talk may have stayed quiet, but they hurt for you because they wish they had taken action themselves when they were younger, and they may have given up long ago. Parents everywhere want their children to have a better life than they did, however, and like as not, your parents wish you were thinner.

Those of us who've lost one or both parents can only go by what we know they tried to get us to do. My father made reserved, respectful comments now and then about hoping I would take off some excess poundage. I had a conversation with him back in the last century about his earlier life. We had just looked at some old B&W photographs, one of them showing him standing with me and my mother out on our front sidewalk when I was about four years old. Daddy was quite large in the photo. He was 6' 2", so he could carry more weight than the average man (about 5' 10"). But he was over

300 lbs. in that picture. He waxed regretful as we talked about the day that picture was taken, and he said he was ashamed that he had gotten that way, and he said that my mother had risen to the occasion and had helped him to lose almost a hundred pounds over the next two or three years. How did he do it, I asked. "A lot of lettuce, son, a lot of lettuce," he replied.

My father never got thin, per se; he hadn't ever been thin as a boy, either. He did get to about 215 lbs., however, and maintained that weight within a few pounds for the rest of his 83 years.

I don't have to wonder what my parents would want me to do about my weight. I know they would want me trim and fit. My getting that way was the only way to honor them in this regard.

VI.

AFTER FAT MAKES YOU MISERABLE, THEN IT KILLS YOU. BUMMER.

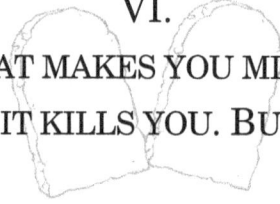

The Original 6th Commandment:
THOU SHALT NOT KILL (EXODUS 20:13).

Some people think the original 6th Commandment prohibits any kind of killing. It does not. Twenty-five verses after Exodus says, "Thou shalt not kill," it says, "He that smiteth a man, so that he die, shall be surely put to death" (Exodus 21:12). Later, other discussions ensue about accidental killings, crimes of passion, justifiable war, and so on. What the 6th Commandment prohibits is murder, and the Hebrew word in the original text confirms this.

Suicide is nothing more than murdering yourself, and it is covered by the 6th Commandment. God's intention was that his people should respect the value of human life and not end a human life for reasons other than just ones.

Let's be very calm, frank, and honest with ourselves for a moment—I hope you've been doing that throughout this book so far. Obesity increases a person's risk of developing the diseases that often result in premature death. There's no escaping this fact. It's true that not every person who is grossly overweight develops diabetes or heart disease or high blood pressure, some of the major conditions that bring lower life expectancy with them, but people who weigh far more than they should, develop those diseases much more often than their thinner counterparts.

The breakpoint, we might say, in the greatest risk of mortality from being overweight comes when a person becomes morbidly obese. Morbid obesity is defined variously, with some monetarily interested parties (bariatric surgeons, for instance) saying it's when you're only 20% over your ideal weight (which also varies). A man who ought to weigh 185 lbs for his height and age (to use our previous illustration) would therefore be morbidly obese if he were just 231 lbs. I think that definition is low. Another authority says that being morbidly obese is when you weigh 100 lbs. or more over your ideal weight (285 lbs. for our example man), or have a BMI (Body Mass Index) of 40 or more, or if you already have some of the typical obesity-related conditions.[15]

Let's just say that before I followed my own *Thin Commandments,* I was morbidly obese. I didn't really look *that* bad, since I am almost 6' 3" and have a large frame. I carried myself erectly and walked briskly, as I had all my life, and that gave me some illusion of not being very much overweight. (There's a "fat walk," which actors learn, that can even make a thin person look overweight.) But there was no hiding my profile. I had come to the point at which

---

[15]Highland Hospital, "What is Morbid Obesity?" University of Rochester Highland Hospital (2015), *https://www.urmc.rochester.edu/highland/ bariatric-surgery-center/questions/morbid-obesity.aspx*, Accessed June 4, 2015.

I could no longer suck in my gut and hold reserve air in my chest and look like I was just burly. I was fat. I was more than a little fat. I was obese.

So far, I had not developed any of the common conditions associated with morbid obesity.[16] An injury to my knee revealed I had some arthritis, but I had no symptoms. My BP was in the normal range until I had to go to the doctor for something, when it went up for psychological reasons (doctors call this "white-coat syndrome").

What I did experience, however, were other inconveniences: when I bent over to tie my shoes, which I could still do fairly easily, I cut off my aortic flow and quickly began to be short of breath; when I needed to run a short distance, it winded me; and getting up from deep sofas was hard. I realized these things weren't going to get better except by addressing their cause, which was excess weight. I also realized that I was likely to develop some of the classic conditions that went along with being obese if I stayed that way. I came to the sober conclusion that I was in the process of killing myself. I just didn't know how soon it was going to happen.

A defensive person will think, Well, it might not happen at all. I might not get diabetes, or heart disease, or high blood pressure or anything. He might say to himself, I know people who weighed 300 lbs. and lived to 100, and even then they died in a skydiving accident. —I'm exaggerating, but

---

[16]Type 2 diabetes, hypertension (high blood pressure), heart disease, sleep apnea, gastroesophageal reflux disease (GERD), gallstones, and osteoarthritis are often mentioned.

you know what I'm saying. If you don't want to do something, you can always find evidence to support your objection.

Yes, I know people who lived to ripe old ages who were overweight. I also know some who died at 90 who smoked, or died at 85 (still well over the average life expectancy) who were alcoholics—these habits carry life-threatening dangers with them, too. But that's what we call anecdotal evidence, and in scientific matters, which is what we should be concerned with here, anecdotal evidence doesn't mean much.

It's kind of like the fellow who says he doesn't believe in wearing seat belts because he knew a guy who had a wreck, his car caught on fire, and he burned to death because he couldn't get out of his seatbelt. Or it's like the parents who have been frightened by something they've read and have decided they aren't going to get their children immunized by vaccination. Never mind the fact that the benefits of vaccination greatly outweigh the risks of adverse effects from vaccinations themselves, these parents choose to take the risk, because they know someone, or heard a terrible story about someone, who was paralyzed by a vaccination.

Suppose you are in a passageway you have to go through, and at the end are two doors. Let's say you know the door on the right leads to an alley where you have a 25% chance of being beaten, robbed, and killed before being able to escape at the other end of it. The door on the left leads to a short street where there is only a 1% chance that anything bad will happen to you. Which door would you choose to go through?

Choosing to remain obese is choosing the door to what will, in all probability, be a shorter and more problem filled life. When being out of breath, getting tired faster (not just from growing older), being limited in what clothes you can wear, having to go to the doctor more often, having to take pills for this and that condition related to obesity, etc., have taken their toll and have cost you lots of money and made you miserable, the likelihood is that one of those conditions will enlarge or become exacerbated, or you will have a sudden episode with one of them that simply takes you out of this world. Bummer.

The 6th *Thin Commandment* is really only a blunt statement of truth, but its implication is just a terse restatement of the divine original: Don't kill yourself with your own fork.

VII.
FAT HURTS YOUR LOVE LIFE:
LOVING FOOD IS CHEATING ON YOUR SPOUSE.

The Original 7th Commandment:
THOU SHALT NOT COMMIT ADULTERY (EXODUS 20:14).

Of all the Ten Commandments that modern people have tampered with, ignored, relegated to the dust bin of antiquity, declared irrelevant, or otherwise tried to get around, this one about adultery is still pretty well regarded as valid. You've probably caught on to the fact that I regard all the others as valid, too, but I won't chase that theological rabbit at this point. Suffice it to say that even many atheists believe that it's wrong for someone else to sleep with their husbands or wives. I wonder why? Outside religious circles people don't often use the word "adultery," but simply say their spouses "cheated" on them.

Even those who don't bother to get married don't want to be cheated on. The guy who has slept with probably more than two dozen women, has lived with three, and then decides to live with another, is nevertheless still fornicating with her. But he is offended if he catches her in bed with another man (or woman, these days), even though his significant other, who isn't his wife after all, had a dozen other bed mates herself before him. The guy's reasoning is that he and she decided to live together and it was *implied,* even if it wasn't explicitly stated, that they wouldn't have sex with other people. She cheated.

Even boyfriends and girlfriends "going steady," as my generation used to say, not living together, don't like to be cheated on, which may mean only going out with someone else—no sex involved.

No one likes to be cheated on, especially in a marriage. Readers of this book are likely to be married or to be in some sort of relationship in which they expect faithfulness in their partners. What does being grossly overweight have to do with it?

As the 7th *Thin Commandment* says, fat interferes with your love life.

- Being significantly overweight tends to lower sex drive.
- Being significantly overweight often reduces sexual enjoyment.
- Being significantly overweight usually deteriorates sexual performance.

I don't intend to get too deep into the physiology and psychology of sex. However, the impact that weight has on sex is exactly what the 7th *Thin Commandment* is about. To provide the basic information, let me give you a summary of a WebMD article on the subject.

Cultural pressures, psychological effects and physical

problems associated with obesity often negatively affect a person's sex life. High cholesterol and insulin resistance (connected to type 2 diabetes) affect sexual performance and desire, especially in men. Both conditions inhibit blood flow to the sex organs and are therefore often responsible for ED (erectile dysfunction). Women are affected by the same problem, as their sexual response depends on blood flow to the genitals, also affected in them by fat. Loss of this blood flow deters lubrication, arousal, and orgasmic function.

Psychological problems associated with obesity also interfere. A negative body image tends to depress desire by making one feel unattractive.[17]

Add to these medical and psychological impacts the most obvious deleterious effect of fat on sex. In men, excess weight effectively shortens the length of the penis, and in women a thick layer of fat hampers access to the vagina. The result is more difficult pairing. Many books and articles have been written about dealing with this problem, finding ways and positions to make better sex possible. *How about losing weight?*

The negative impact on a couple's sex life is potentially significant. If the love affair of one or both partners with food is to blame for the interruption or even cessation of their love life with each other, isn't the love of food tantamount to cheating on your spouse?

---

[17]Colette Bouchez, "Better Sex: What's Weight Got to Do with It?" WebMD (2015), *http://www.webmd.com/sex-relationships/features/ sex-and-weight*, Accessed June 4, 2015.

VIII.
DON'T SNEAK FOOD:
YOU WILL WEAR THE EVIDENCE.

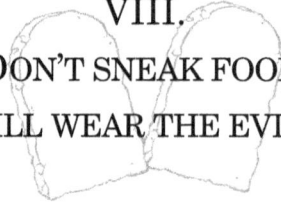

Nothing is more central to the laws of all civilized society than the right of possession. No just government on earth denies people the right to personal property. Some communist and socialist governments restrict ownership of real estate, while democratic republics, like our American system, champion that right. But people everywhere have the right to possess things and they justly expect their governments to protect that right against anyone who would take away those things .

Nothing has ever made me more livid than stealing. I'm sure the feeling goes back into my youth, when I had a bicycle stolen by a neighborhood bully. I recovered it, but the very idea that he would take what was mine was infuriating. Throughout my life from time to time someone has stolen things from me. It never gets easier for me to deal with emotionally.

The Original 8th Commandment was of obvious moral necessity. It isn't right to steal. Most of the time, people don't take your stuff while you're watching; most often, people who steal come when you're not around, sneak into your home or yard, and take something that isn't theirs.

The 8th *Thin Commandment* is a little different. It doesn't tell you not to steal food from others, but not to take it for yourself when you should be leaving it in the pantry, in the freezer, in the refrigerator, in the box, or in the bag or wrapper. You know what those things are.

Sneaking food is interesting. I've done it; we've all done it. You have a little stash of something that's particularly satisfying to you when you're hungry: a bag of candy or a box of cookies, for instance. It's usually sweet, though not always, and it's usually not refrigerated, because the whole point is to stash it somewhere that no one else knows about and to access it when no one's watching. You can sneak treats from the fridge, too, and it can be something as innocuous as crackers and cheese, though it's usually not celery or raw carrots—what fun is that?

The problem is that when you're eating less, you get hungry sooner between meals, and you go looking for something to eat surreptitiously. As long as you are uninterrupted, you can continue to dip into the stash, sneaking bite after bite, until any progress you made that day by eating less at meals is undone by snacking.

Snacks themselves are not bad: sometimes you need a snack to avoid indulging at an upcoming meal. What you snack on, however, makes a big difference, especially if you don't intend to minimize the impact by getting "just a little something." Diet experts tell us to choose "healthy snacks," which they usually define as fruits and raw vegetables. I'm not going to dismiss that suggestion out of hand; I happen to like celery and raw carrots, and cutting a fresh apple and enjoying it while watching TV is sometimes exactly what the doctor called for (who, if the axiom is accurate, I should be able to keep away from me if I eat enough apples).

However, I'm not going to suggest that you eliminate snacks, or that you never snack on chocolate covered English toffee, which happens to be a favorite of mine. What I am going to suggest is that you eat your snacks in front of someone else as a witness. Sometimes just that sense of accountability implicit in another person's presence is enough to curb your indulgence. If you live alone, your dog or cat won't do as a witness (Sorry), so you'll just have to discipline yourself.

I'm also going to suggest that you calculate the impact on your daily intake, and limit yourself to what will not cancel out your otherwise lower intake of food. If that means counting calories, then do it if you must, but it need not mean anything more than that you develop a sense for what level of snacking will be negligible. That witness may be able to help you more than you realize.

I happen to know, for instance, that if I eat a small breakfast, a nearly harmless lunch like a vegetable salad, and a sensible supper, I can eat a few pieces of toffee mid evening and still make progress on my weight loss. The ability to enjoy the things I like keeps me from feeling deprived and eliminates the fear that strikes in the heart of dieters everywhere that they will never be able to enjoy sweet or rich foods again. What is our key to losing weight and keeping it off? *It's amounts—that's all!*

Back in 1983 the Frito-Lay company, makers of Lay's Potato Chips, ran a series of ads with the slogan, "Bet you can't eat just one." It was a very successful campaign because it latched onto a weakness we all have: indulgence. Sit down with a bag of chips or your favorite snack in a bulk amount, with nothing much to do but watch TV, and you're a good candidate for a bout with hedonic hyperphagia, the technical term for eating for pleasure, without hunger and often to excess.[18]

One of the best remedies, if not the very best, to attacks of snacking indulgence is to snack only in the presence of that witness I recommended. If you have a mate, just bring the bag or box into the common room and sit down with it there. When you sneak off by yourself to have a snack, it usually means you are trying to deceive someone. It could be your spouse or significant other, but it could be merely yourself.

Human beings have a fascinating capacity to believe that they can hide things from themselves. If there are others around, we may hide our private indulgences from them, but if there's no one else to deceive, we may engage in simply deceiving ourselves. It's almost like we pretend that if no one else sees it, it didn't happen. When it comes to sneaking food, the problem is that we will likely display the

---

[18]Kayt Sukel, "The science of 'Bet you can't eat just one'" (BigThink, 2013) *http://bigthink.com/world-in-mind/bet-you-cant-eat-just-one,* Accessed June 5, 2015.

results of frequent and excessive snacking in the most public sort of way: we'll get, or stay, fat.

The most obvious evidence that our diets aren't working is our failure to make progress. The pants still won't fit. The belt can't be pulled tighter and may have to be adjusted to the next hole out. The shirt or blouse buttons are taught. We go to wearing shirts or tops out rather than tucked in. Our faces don't have the contours they used to.

When we sneak food, we're probably not stealing from someone else, but we're stealing from ourselves. We're stealing the enjoyment of life that belongs to the more mobile, more active, more able, more flexible, more healthy person we could be. Further, we're not fooling anybody. Everybody knows we indulge ourselves. Even if we make a great show of eating a salad at lunch out with the staff or say No to dessert or second helpings at dinner, if we remain greatly overweight and don't change, everyone knows we're eating in private what we self-righteously deny ourselves in public.

IX.

DON'T LIE TO YOURSELF: YOU DON'T
NEED IT; YOU JUST WANT IT.

The Original 9ᵗʰ Commandment:
THOU SHALT NOT BEAR FALSE WITNESS
AGAINST THY NEIGHBOUR (EXODUS 20:16)

The Original 9ᵗʰ Commandment against lying was expressed in terms that focused on those untruths that hurt other people—false testimony before a judge, tall tales that malign someone, and so on. The New Testament certainly reflects the idea that lying in general is wrong: "Lie not one to another" (Colossians 3:9). Lying almost always hurts the one lied about and the one lied to.

We won't dwell on the possible circumstances where lying would be right. The classic example is a Nazi who asks a German householder, "Do you have Jews here?" to which the householder says, "No," when in fact there is a family living in the attic. What we're concerned with here is the kind of untruth we are tempted to tell *ourselves*.

The 9ᵗʰ *Thin Commandment* warns us against self-deception. Every person is at his most persuasive when speaking or reasoning to himself. We can all talk ourselves into things that no one else ever could. And we're good listeners, too! We can have both sides of the classic conversation with ourselves where the little angels, or our better selves, are sitting on our right shoulders and the little devils, or our mischievous selves, are sitting on the left. With temptations about food, the way it usually goes is that the voice on the left says, "I really need something to eat," and the right says, "No you don't; you just *want* it." After that, who wins is usually a product of how long we let the conversation go on. The longer we debate with ourselves whether we're going to eat or eat more, the more likely we are to give in. The shorter the conversation is, the more likely our wiser selves are to prevail.

Baseball statistics from 1988 onward show that after four pitches have been thrown to any player at bat, the batter has a greater and greater chance of getting a hit (or a walk) as opposed to making an out. During a game, a hopeful hometown play-by-play man may say of a deepening pitch count at a critical moment, "The advantage goes to the batter."

In the struggle you wage with yourself over snacking, consider yourself the pitcher. You're doing your best from the mound to pitch the benefits of your diet plan to yourself at the plate (pun intended). Again and again you try to convince yourself to stick to the plan, and again and again the adverse you at the plate says, "One more won't hurt." And one more after that, and so on. The longer this at-bat continues, the more likely the you who has the plate will win and the you who is pitching his best to eat less will lose.

End the contest quickly. Put the snack back, Jack.

X.

IT'S NOT FOOD THAT TEMPTS YOU:
IT'S YOU, ALWAYS THINKING ABOUT IT.

The Original 10ᵗʰ Commandment:
THOU SHALT NOT COVET (EXODUS 20:17).

One way to look at the Ten Commandments' prohibition of coveting is that if you were able to follow it faithfully, you wouldn't disobey some of the other Commandments either. You wouldn't want to work seven days a week (the 4ᵗʰ Commandment); you wouldn't want to do what your parents wished you wouldn't do (the 5ᵗʰ); you wouldn't want what you might get by someone else's being dead (the 6ᵗʰ) you wouldn't want somebody else's wife or husband (the 7ᵗʰ); and you wouldn't want other people's stuff (the 8ᵗʰ). Coveting—yearning in an inordinate way to possess something that belongs to someone else—is at the root of many another evil.

The 10ᵗʰ *Thin Commandment* is an application of the original. Spending all your time thinking about food constitutes inordinate desire—a excessive preoccupation with eating.

Think about obsessing over food as being like coveting what isn't yours *yet*. It may belong to you if you bought it from the grocery store, but it's not in your mouth *yet*. It isn't part of your body *yet*. Often, after imagining our next meal all morning or afternoon, when we have it before us we may find ourselves stuffing it down so fast that we don't take time to enjoy it. Savoring food is a joy built into the very fact that what is edible to us has a rich breadth of taste and texture. We were meant to enjoy what we have to do—eat— not simply to get as much of it as we can into our bellies as fast as possible.

A particularly gross and *literally* gross character in the *Austin Powers* films was a morbidly obese villain with cannibalistic tendencies. Hoping to capitalize on the popularity of *Austin Powers* with a certain segment of the population, DirecTV® produced some ads with this character and the Mini-Me character from those same films. In the ads, the fat villain leered hungrily at Mini-Me and used a line from the films: "Come on, get in my belly!"

Personally, I found the concept bizarre. I had not seen the films, their not being my taste in entertainment. But the jarring idea of a tremendously fat person ordering a diminutive creature to hop in his mouth and be eaten, stuck in a corner of my brain. It came out when I thought of this 10th *Thin Commandment*. Thinking about food all the time creates ongoing temptation. Temptation encouraged by obsessive consideration leads to indulgence, and the rapid, often ravenous consumption of food once it's in sight bespeaks inordinate desire: covetousness.

We often tell ourselves that food tempts us. It doesn't have to be food that's "bad" for us; it can be food that virtually no health nut condemns. If, because we've been obsessing over food, we're inclined to load up our plates with much more of that food than we need, however (Remember the triple-decker plates at the buffet?), we're being tempted. The question is, by whom or what?[19]

You know the answer, of course. Food doesn't tempt. Living beings tempt. Unless you're with someone who is trying to get you to stuff yourself, it's you who is tempting yourself. Stop saying "I was tempted." The passive voice in that sentence means the speaker doesn't want to admit who was doing the tempting. You and I tempt ourselves with food. It looks tempting, to be sure, but any actual temptation comes from our own minds, and possibly hearts.

Psychologists have a term for our blaming the food for the temptation: projection. Projection is a defense mechanism that involves taking our own unacceptable qualities or feelings and ascribing them to others,[20] in this case, to food personified. Those whose religious views incorporate the idea of the intricate involvement of a personal tempter in every person's life, all day long, may want to offer a counter argument here that Satan may be tempting them to overeat. I won't make this portion of the

---

[19]I reject the notion that foods with some ingredient that a nutritionist somewhere disapproves of are therefore inherently bad for us. The adage of moderation in all things applies. Foods that are truly bad for us in all likelihood have not been allowed by government to be sold. Everything else is subject to moderation. Before the Italians popularized them, tomatoes were bad for you: they were presumed to be poisonous. Thank God for rebels who ate them.

[20]Kendra Cherry, "Defense Mechanisms," *About.com* (2015) *http://psychology.about.com/od/theoriesofpersonality/ss/defensemech_7.htm,* Accessed June 5, 2015.

book a theological treatise, but any serious study of the Bible indicates that neither Satan nor any one of his henchmen is involved in every temptation. In fact, a key Bible verse on the subject says, "Every man is tempted, when he is drawn away *of his own lust,* and enticed" (James 1:14, emphasis mine). We have enough ability to tempt ourselves without always being hounded by some separate, evil entity.

The bottom line is that we need to put food in its place. It is necessary. As a blessing, it's also enjoyable. It should be eaten with celebration and thankfulness, in a responsible and controlled manner. It's not a god to be worshiped or that will control us (the 1st and 2nd *Thin Commandments)*; it's not a thing to be loved more than the people in our lives (the 5th and 7th *Thin Commandments)*; it's not to be done without ever taking a rest (the 4th *Thin Commandment)*; and it should sustain and enrich our lives, not limit and destroy them (all the rest of the *Thin Commandments)*.

The way to keep all these *Thin Commandments* is to learn the discipline of eating less. When you eat less, you will lose weight. *It's amounts, amounts, amounts! That's all.*

6
A Challenge for the New You
Setting a Wonderful Goal

I don't know who is reading this book. I suspect the average person interested in the title would be someone with a mate, someone over thirty, perhaps a good bit more. In fact, I suspect that the average reader was thin, or at least not morbidly obese, earlier in life, but will have gained a lot of weight over a good many years, and will be looking for some way to get back to how he/she looked a long time ago. I'm going to offer a turn-of-phrase motto for that average reader, believing that it will be useful to others as well, with only a little amendment and adjustment. Here it is:

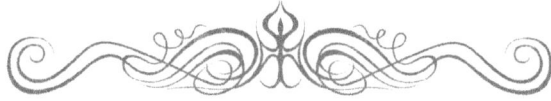

I cannot gain youth
once I've lost it,
but I can lose
what I gained
while I was
losing it.

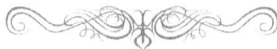

Notice how the short motto gets thinner as it goes down. So will you as your weight goes down.

As I entered my 60s, I went through a time when I was frequently and deeply nostalgic. I had an enjoyable childhood and youth, good parents, nice places to live, and a good education. My first career was fulfilling in many ways, stressful in others. My children were a delight and my wife a joy to live with. Though my second career, entered in my 50s, has been greatly rewarding, and though my children, now adults, are two to be proud of, and though I enjoy my hobbies and activities and my life, all around, still I am nostalgic. Among the books I have written I have frequently dealt with the subject of time travel; sometimes I greatly wish I could revisit my life forty or fifty years ago, if not to undo or redo something, then just to experience it again.

One of the things I found myself wishing for as much or more than anything about my past, was to be as light as I was in my early twenties. That's an unrealistic goal for many people, especially if they were very, very thin. With the combined effect of age on skin and the result of having acquired a lot of extra weight, most people who weigh significantly more than they did at 20 or 25 will not be able to achieve their exact youthful weight. We would be surprised, however, at how close to it we could come, if we fixed our eyes on the goal, committed ourselves to reaching it, and followed this one overarching rule: eat less.

You can't go back in time and gain your youth, but the pounds you gained while you were losing your youth, you can lose. That alone will make you feel much younger. The *Thin Commandments* are the truths that can guide you, warn you, remind you, teach you, correct you, and inspire you as you set out on your journey to recover—or uncover for the first time—the slimmer person you can be.

www.ingramcontent.com/pod-product-compliance
Lightning Source LLC
Chambersburg PA
CBHW030026290326

41934CB00005B/511